Spontaneous Joyful Natural Birth

A Collection of Birth Stories and Guide to the
Beauty and Benefits of Delivering Your Baby Naturally

Natasha Panzer

Spontaneous Joyful Natural Birth

A Collection of Birth Stories and Guide to the
Beauty and Benefits of Delivering Your Baby Naturally

Praeclarus Press, LLC

2504 Sweetgum Lane

Amarillo, Texas 79124 USA

806-367-9950

www.PraeclarusPress.com

DISCLAIMER

The information contained in this publication is advisory only and is not intended to replace sound clinical judgment or individualized patient care. The author disclaims all warranties, whether expressed or implied, including any warranty as the quality, accuracy, safety, or suitability of this information for any particular purpose.

ISBN: 978-1-939807-79-3

Dedication

I dedicate this book to my children, Sofia and Emmett.

You never cease to amaze, delight, and inspire me.

"Story is such a powerful way to transmit the beauty, power, strength and love in birth. Natasha Panzer imparts those elements with this powerful book that once read a pregnant momma has a good chance at the natural birth her baby wants. These amazing stories remind me of what my dear friend Sister MorningStar says, "What one woman can do, all women can do." Sister also tells us, "Story is more powerful than fact." This book will help us change the birth paradigm and give birthing women the respect they deserve. Give one to every pregnant woman you meet!"

Jan Tritten, Midwife, founder and editor-in-chief of *Midwifery Today* magazine

Acknowledgments

My own personal experiences with the delicacy and power of pregnancy and birth have solidified my deep admiration for the profession of midwifery. I am immeasurably grateful for the support I have received from the Connecticut Childbirth and Women's Center and its incredible director, Catherine Parisi, MSN, CNM, a remarkable individual I have chosen to highlight in this book. She and her outstanding staff have seen me through my three very different pregnancies, and this book is my way of saying thank you for helping me bring my children into this world feeling supported and empowered. I also want to especially thank Catherine Gallagher, CNM, without whom I am not sure I could have achieved the birth of my dreams. By encouraging me to read *Ina May Gaskin's Guide to Childbirth*, I was opened up to a whole new realm of birth possibilities and finally began to realize that the kind of birth I had desired from the start was possible.

Thank you to all the incredible mothers, fathers, midwives, and doulas who shared their experiences for the book. Your words will help others find the encouragement to trust their strength, believe in the process, and stay the course. Together, we will help improve birth one great story at a time!

I want to thank my good friends Kathryn Nixon and Laura Drossman for their time, encouragement, advice, and editorial assistance. Without you two, this book may never have made it past the proposal stage.

Eternal thanks to Hale Publishing for believing in the importance of these stories. Special thanks to Katherine Kendall-Tackett for giving a first timer a chance and to Janet Rourke for your patience and your guidance throughout the editorial process.

Thank you to my family and friends, especially Kristen, who gave me the initial push and my dear sister-in-law Jennifer O'Hara, who kept my children safe and happy through all the hours I could not be with them as I worked on this project. I am also very grateful to Jennifer Taney Panzer for helping me with some of the photographs in this book.

I would also like to express my sincere appreciation for the kind words and encouragement I received from both Ina May Gaskin and Jan Tritten in support of this project.

To my husband Justin, who encouraged my birth choices, and helped me feel like the most powerful woman on the planet after our incredible water birth, I give my deepest gratitude. I love you.

And a tremendous thank you to my wonderful children. I will be forever grateful for your patience during this writing and editing process. While I always prefer to be with you, the importance of the project demanded our mutual sacrifice. Emmett: you were the best birth partner a mama could ever ask for! Together we had one wild ride. Thank you for enlightening me! Sofia—your birth, no less enlightening, forged the way! May you grow up fully realizing your capabilities, strength, and incredible beauty. I love you both so very much!

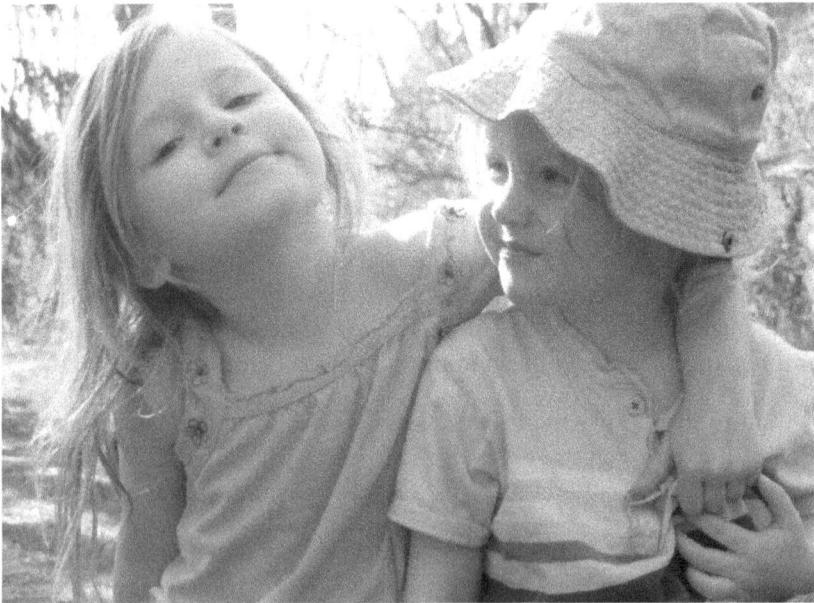

Table of Contents

Introduction

Why This Book Needed to be Written

Women have been cajoled into accepting the birthing agendas of others for far too long. It is time for women to take back their right to choose the kind of birth they desire, and it is time for our country as a whole to adopt logical, civilized birth practices, which have been proven through research to be best for mother and baby.

The culture of birthing in the United States is now dominated by medical interventions; so much so, that natural childbirth is often regarded as the alternative rather than the normal means for birthing a healthy baby. Interventions, such as inducing labor with synthetic oxytocin and administering epidurals, have become so commonplace that many women have lost sight of the adverse effects these interventions can have on mother and child. Even more alarming, the rate of scheduled cesareans continues to rise, and many women falsely believe that vaginal birth after cesarean is always a dangerous choice, when in fact it can be the safest and most rewarding conclusion to a healthy pregnancy. Midwives in America are still fighting in many states for the right to do their jobs and support women through labor and delivery; and those who have found a way to work are often limited by illogical hospital regulations and the threat of malpractice. Women who desire to birth their babies in a safe, gentle, and natural way and those who have dedicated their lives to assist in that process should be supported and not marginalized.

Time and time again, laboring mothers are being asked to succumb to medical interventions "for the sake of their babies" without medical necessity and are suffering consequences not clearly explained to them. Many women are being subjected to interventions they do not want or consent to. Where are the ethics? What ever happened to "first do no harm"? Labor inducing drugs, drugs that augment contractions, pain-numbing medications, electro fetal monitoring, and C-sections are being pushed on laboring mothers regularly. Why? Not because they make the laboring mother more comfortable or are necessarily safer. On the contrary, these interventions make moving around during labor nearly impossible and inhibit a women from moving instinctually to naturally ease the intensity of her contractions. They prohibit women from birthing in an upright position and benefiting from gravity. Oftentimes, women are restricted from drinking or eating, a practice now believed by many to only weaken a women, who if allowed, will eat and drink only what she needs to retain the energy necessary to birth her baby on her own strength.

So, why has our society, which clearly places so much emphasis on the health and wellbeing of its children, regularized a style of birthing that is not the safest or healthiest means for either party directly involved? Regrettably, too many have put their faith in medicine and technology and have undervalued the ability and strength of the female body and mind. We, collectively, have lost track of several simple facts—the female body is designed for birth, women are strong, and babies born spontaneously, without medical interventions, thrive. We have been conditioned to fear the pain of birth, and we, too often, lack the support we need to conquer that fear. Fortunately, I found my way past my own fears to experience the amazing natural birth of my son in 2009, an experience which opened my eyes. I learned natural birth was an incredibly powerful, life-changing experience that needed more promotion before it became truly extinct. I learned that natural birth, while wonderful, magical, and transformative, was also very, very normal. Not a very exciting word, but an important one. My experience certainly inspired me, but the amazing collection of first-hand birth experiences I have assembled for this book and the supplemental information I have included give my message the additional support I needed to show that natural birth is possible in a myriad of settings, even hospitals ... and it is worthwhile.

Women who plan to birth their babies naturally will find the encouragement to do so in many places. Much of our understanding of the birth process begins to form very early in our lives as we first hear stories from our family about birth and are exposed to our first images of birth. Children who witness the birth of animals often have positive feelings about birth, realizing it is normal and possible to birth without interventions. My own positive associations with birth began as a young child, when I first viewed powerful images of positive, natural birth experiences.

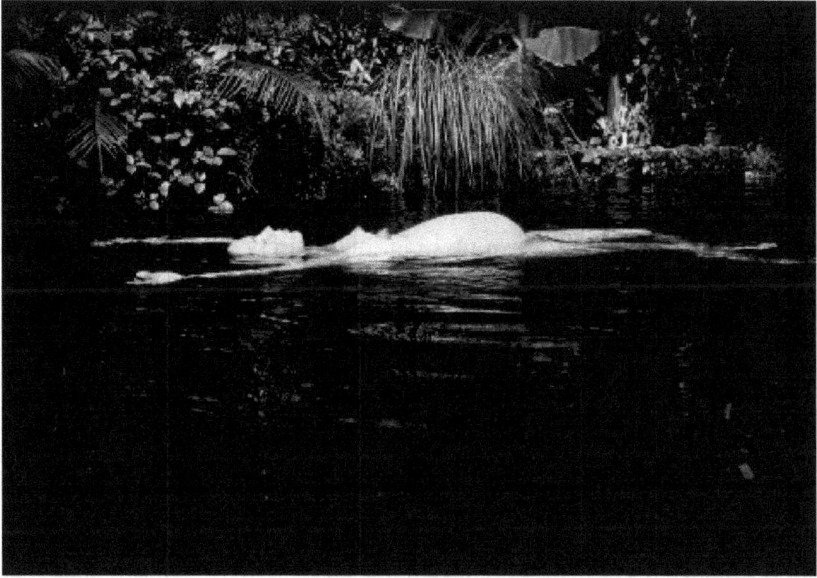

Photo courtesy of Neil Schwartz

I was brought up watching "natural birth" slide shows my father created during his foray into photojournalism in the early 1970s. One series he shot in south Florida shows a woman laboring in a beautiful, tropical pond, floating peacefully with a plump pregnant belly, as she prepares for her birth.

She then moves into her home, seeking warmth from a shower, and births her baby with her own two hands, gently and peacefully as her husband and a friend look on.

The mother then puts the baby to her breast and proceeds outside to the hand-made birthing chair her husband has crafted and painted with ornate floral designs, which waits for her in their garden. There she, seemingly painlessly, births the placenta while nursing her newborn. To this day, my father still loves to tell the story of this shoot and marvels how the woman strapped the baby to her body in a wrap and bicycled over to his house later that evening to view the pictures of her birth.

As a child I was slightly embarrassed when my father dragged his "naked lady slide show" out proudly for our dinner party guests, but I realize now that these images helped to form my conception that birthing could be very beautiful and should not be feared. This woman, who chose to birth out of the hospital, squatting in her own home shower, didn't look like a renegade bad-ass scoffing at the norm, nor did she look like a risk-taker. She was calm, even in the throws of labor, and the pictures portray birth as a magical moment that was very free, yet under the control of the laboring woman. This woman had a vision of what her birth should be and made it happen. She defied the modern medical practices of her day and took matters into her own hands. Even as a child, I was struck by how peaceful birth could be. The seed was planted.

I also grew up watching the black and white slide show of my own birth— my mother's labor, my crowning head, my first cry. This, I have to admit, was a little harder to sit through. Seeing my mother's under-carriage on a five-by-five screen, while surrounded by visiting relatives, was a little rough. I would squint and wince, but eventually I saw it all. My mother sat upright in the hospital bed in what looked to be a very dimly lit room. She was knitting and her legs donned knee-high woolen socks as her feet rested in the stirrups. I pondered the weirdness of this birth. Knee-highs in the middle of June? Knitting during labor? She never looked like she was in pain in any of the pictures, and I know she did not take any pain medications. This was another birth that did not seem to follow the popular refrain that having a baby hurt. If mom could do it, so could I.

The birth I had in mind had been shaped by these images, as well as from a few "alternative" birth stories I saw on television while I was first pregnant. One birth, which really made me reconsider the importance of birth location, showed footage of a women birthing in a warm tidal pool in Hawaii. She and her husband had built a camping platform on the side of this tidal pool, believing it to be the perfect birthing location, and documented the entire event with a camcorder on a tripod. When labor began the women spent much of her time in the warm salty water, bending and resting in various positions. When the baby emerged, it looked as if it actually swam to the surface. The father clamped the cord, they waited for the pulsations to cease, and he made the cut. Mother, father, and healthy baby relaxed for the rest of the day on their private platform, embracing and enjoying the moment. While I was not about to erect a campsite and birth outdoors, I thought this water birth looked very pleasant and beautiful. I had my doubts about the safety of the location, but I felt happy for the couple that they were able to see their vision through.

Another television program opened up my eyes to a really empowering element I wanted to try during my own birth. In the episode a young woman was laboring in a hospital with her mother by her side. When it came time to push the baby out, her doctor directed her to bend over, reach down, and pull the baby up onto her chest, once his head and upper body were clear. She did just that and smiled heartily as the nurses suctioned the baby's airways, while he lay on her chest and she admired him. It was thrilling. She delivered her own baby. How powerful, I thought. What an awesome way to begin bonding.

With all these images rattling around in my head and with his own idea of a bucolic hospital-free setting, my husband and I began to build the vision of our ideal birth. We discussed the possibility of a home birth for a while. One of our sister-in-laws had three of her four children at home with the assistance of a midwife. Justin, my husband, had been staying at his brother's home during one of these births and was very impressed. Still, I was reluctant, and we decided a nearby free-standing birth center was the best choice for us. While we learned first-hand that there are no guarantees in pregnancy and childbirth, we discovered that our original hopes to birth out of a hospital, in a safe, supported, encouraging environment was attainable if we stayed focused on our ideal birth.

Every woman has an opportunity to create a birth plan that is personal and meaningful. These plans are shaped by what we see and what we hear throughout our lives. I was fortunate to have seen enough positive images and heard enough positive messages about natural birth to believe in the process and create a plan that paved the way to my own incredible natural birth. Still, I believe the world needs more of these positive images and encouraging stories. Women need to see more beautiful, peaceful, and empowering images of birth to believe in it. Women need to read more positive first-hand accounts to realize that birth does not have to be something to fear. The culture of birth needs to change, and I believe that change can happen, with each amazing birth story that is shared.

When I decided to put this book together, I reached out to the natural birthing community, posting ads in birth centers and on like-minded blogs and Facebook pages, asking if any women would like to share their stories. The response was incredible. I became fast friends with women all over the United States and two women in New Zealand who wanted to be a part of the project. Time and again, I was reminded of the importance of these stories and was encouraged to press forward and see the project to completion.

The majority of the stories I received for this collection highlight the unique care and support one will experience when they elect to birth in a free-standing birth center. Interestingly, while I posted advertisements in almost every state, I received multiple contributions from a few specific areas; communities which clearly have a very strong connection to their birth centers. Because of the tremendous response from the clients of The Connecticut Childbirth & Women's Center in Danbury, Connecticut, the Mountain Midwifery Center in Englewood, Colorado, and the Morning

Star Birth Center in St. Louis Park, Minnesota, these three centers are specifically featured in this book. They, along with the other well-regarded established birth centers highlighted on these pages, stand as excellent examples of how the wellness model of pregnancy and birth care is thriving in some areas of our country.

While a free-standing birth center is a fantastic option for a healthy woman who has enjoyed a normal pregnancy, they are still few and far between. Most women in this country are still birthing in traditional hospital maternity wards. While the majority of American woman are opting for a medicalized birth, many are still determined to let their body do its work without interventions, albeit in the hospital. Several of the stories in this book show how positive natural birthing experiences, while challenging, are still possible within hospitals when the mother and her supporters stick to their convictions. And for those courageous women who desire to birth vaginally after a C-section, the hospital is the safest choice. I was astounded by the VBAC stories I received for the book. I am especially proud to share the stories of the three women who overcame their fears, lovingly prepared their bodies and minds for a remarkable challenge, and persevered.

The final topic of the book, home birth, ignites powerful opinions at each end of the issue. For those who believe birth is a dangerous prospect, home birth is frightening. For those who understand the process of birth and are educated about the true risks, home birth can seem like a very normal, logical choice for a healthy woman. I have chosen to include two categories of home birth: planned and unexpected.

Birth is unpredictable. There is much that a laboring woman cannot control. Still, a woman can control where she chooses to birth; she can control who she chooses to support her; she can control her birth plan; and she can take action to see the plan through.

With this book I hope to encourage women to make mindful birthing choices. I hope to encourage women to carefully choose a birth attendant who will honor their wishes. With this book I hope to strongly encourage moms-to-be to consider using midwives and doulas to support them throughout their pregnancy and birth. I also wish to commend obstetricians who honor their patients' requests to birth naturally and encourage those who have lost sight of women's innate ability to birth naturally to reassess their influence. A healthy woman who has experienced a normal pregnancy, spontaneously goes into labor, and is allowed to labor naturally does not need saving, she needs support.

I hope this book helps expectant women realize that an unmedicated birth is something worth striving for and something worth fighting for. Most of all, I hope my story, and the other stories in this book, will encourage women to believe in their strength, to ask more questions about their birthing options, to embrace the challenges of labor and birth, and to joyfully pursue the natural, beautiful, transformative birth they deserve.

Part I

The Birth Center Experience

1

Birth Centers

Women who are healthy and wish to birth in a supported, family-centered environment should consider the birth center model of care. While birth centers are starting to grow in numbers in the United States, they have yet to become a standard consideration for the majority of pregnant mothers because many women are simply unsure what a birth center is, what they offer, or where to find one. If there was more awareness of the incredible, individualized attention women enjoy at birth centers, there would, no doubt, be far more of them. The American Association of Birth Centers describes them like this:

> A birth center is a home-like facility, existing within a health care system with a program of care designed in a wellness model of pregnancy and birth. Birth centers are guided by principles of prevention, sensitivity, safety, appropriate medical intervention, and cost effectiveness. Birth centers provide family-centered care for healthy women, before, during, and after normal pregnancy, labor, and birth (2010, p.1).

Most birth centers offer comprehensive gynecological care, allowing women to build strong bonds with their care providers well before they are even pregnant.

No two birth centers are exactly alike. Some birth centers are actually attached to hospitals, yet offer a more natural, low-tech birthing experience. Free-standing birth centers are not attached to hospitals, but are nearby in case obstetric intervention or neonatal care is required. Birth centers are most often directed and operated by certified nurse midwives and sometimes work with the support and cooperation of a particular obstetrician or obstetric group. Birth centers offer women personalized, supportive care in a very comfortable, home-like space. Free-standing birth centers are licensed and follow the standards of care established by the National Association of Childbearing Centers (NACC).

Birth centers usually offer a choice of birthing rooms, many equipped with Jacuzzi tubs or inflatable tubs for relaxing during labor and water birth. Most birth centers have a variety of support tools to assist during labor and birth, like birthing stools, birthing balls, Rebozo wraps, rocking chairs, and comfortable beds. The midwives have all the necessary supplies and equipment at the birth center to assist you during your normal delivery and are well trained to recognize when transfer to the hospital is needed.

Birth centers offer a unique opportunity for mothers to experience continuous, individualized, encouraging care. Birth centers are incredibly positive places, staffed by supportive individuals who truly believe in a woman's innate ability to birth naturally and will allow you to take the lead in your birthing experience. If you are healthy, have experienced a normal pregnancy, and truly wish to avoid unnecessary medical interventions, a birth center is a terrific option to consider.

If you choose to birth at a birth center, you will be cared for primarily by midwives. The modern midwife is well trained in natural, low-tech techniques to support women through pregnancy, labor, and delivery, and has a vast knowledge and breadth of experience to be able to support women in a variety of settings, including in their homes, in birth centers, or in hospitals. Midwives sometimes choose to focus their practice in a particular environment. For instance, some midwives specialize in home birth, while others choose to work solely in free-standing birth centers. The profession of midwifery has come a long way since its ancient origins.

There are several types of midwives, the two main categories being certified nurse-midwives and direct-entry midwives (which include certified professional midwives).

A certified nurse-midwife ...

Is educated and licensed in the two disciplines of nursing and midwifery. She must pass a national certification examination given by the American College of Nurse-Midwives and must meet strict requirements set forth by (her

"Most women spend more time shopping for jeans than shopping for the right birth attendant. Choosing the right provider and place of birth are key to having a satisfying birthing experience. Prenatal care should be fun, educational, sensitive, and respectful. The best providers realize there is not "one way" to birth a baby, but many ways. Care should be individualized—women are individuals and should be treated accordingly."—Catherine Gallagher, CNM

Connecticut Childbirth & Women's Center

state's) Department of Public Health. She provides comprehensive care in all aspects of women's health. This includes low-risk maternity care, attendance at births, postpartum care, contraceptive counseling, screening and treatment of routine gynecological problems, history and physicals, as well as perimenopausal and postmenopausal consultation (Connecticut Childbirth & Women's Center, 2006).

A direct-entry midwife …

Is an independent practitioner educated in the discipline of midwifery through self-study, apprenticeship, a midwifery school, or a college- or university-based program distinct from the discipline of nursing. A direct-entry midwife is trained to provide the Midwives Model of Care to healthy women and newborns throughout the childbearing cycle primarily in out-of-hospital settings (Midwives' Alliance of North America, 2011).

2

Our Ideal Birth Realized

By Natasha Panzer

Even before I became pregnant for the first time, my husband and I daydreamed about the family we would someday form and envisioned a gentle, natural birth for our babies. We shared the belief that hospitals were not the best places to have a baby and felt very fortunate when we discovered a lovely free-standing birth center not far from our home that we felt would respect our views on birthing and support us through the pregnancy and birth. Today, we have two beautiful children who have certainly surpassed our wildest hopes and dreams, but our journey to creating this family did not flow as smoothly as we thought it would.

To say I was naïve about pregnancy and birth when I first set out to become a mom is a vast understatement. I did not get the pregnancy or birth of my dreams the first go around. In fact, I struck out miserably with a devastating miscarriage that really derailed my spirit. My second pregnancy resulted in the birth of an absolutely fantastic individual, our daughter, Sofia. Sofia is bright, hilarious, gorgeous, and has a wonderfully robust character. She keeps me laughing every day, and I can't imagine this world without the light she gives. Sofia's birth, however, was long, painful, and, at times, scary. Although I had wanted to have Sofia at the birth center, I had to be transferred to the hospital across the street, due to her irregular heart rate. My hospital experience was, I am sorry to say, rather typical, and not in a good way. I underwent a series of medical interventions, most of which I now believe I could have avoided had I been better prepared.

My third pregnancy was trying at times, but the labor and birth were truly exceptional, the sort of experience I wasn't quite sure really was possible until I lived it for myself. My son, Emmett, is proving to be as exceptionally cool as his birth was exceptionally smooth. He is bright like his sister and has been strong and alert from his first day out in the big wide world. The birth of my son awakened strength in me that I had not yet recognized and reaffirmed my belief that birth is a natural process that does not have to be painful or scary.

Emmett's awesome birth was made possible partly through my own resolve, but more so by the support and guidance of three special midwives. When I became pregnant for a third time, I already knew that I would attempt once more to give birth at the Connecticut Childbirth and Women's Center, but I was not quite sure how I was going to avoid ending up in the hospital again, caving to unnecessary interventions. A new midwife at the center named Cathy Gallagher helped to guide me in the right direction to realizing my dream birth.

Cathy Gallagher joined the center in 2008 and from the onset I trusted her implicitly. She exuded nurturing warmth and had obvious concern for the well being of her clients. She was every bit as comforting and caring as the Director of the center, Cathy Parisi, who attended my first birth, had assured. During my first meeting with Cathy Gallagher, I felt very much at ease and described the less than ideal hospital experience I had during my daughter Sofia's birth and my hopes to birth at the center this go around. I expressed my fears that I would need to be transferred to the hospital again, and once more be subjected to what I felt was an inevitable chain of medical interventions. I doubted my own natural ability to birth without medication, but still had a deep desire to do so. Cathy listened to everything I said, and then recommended that I read *Ina May Gaskin's Guide to Childbirth*. I left excited and started to feel a shift in my outlook. I ordered the book that night and eagerly checked the mail each day.

When Ina May's book finally arrived, I dove right in. The book described how Ina May became a midwife along the journey from California to Tennessee with her husband Stephen and a caravan of buses. The descriptions of helpful, natural techniques to ease and augment labor made sense and the personal accounts, written in plain English, proved the effectiveness of various techniques. After reading the book, I realized that a woman could have a good deal of control over her labor and birth if she knew what she wanted, was properly supported, and kept focused. I began to realize the vital role of the birth attendants in making sure the woman's vision was realized. I immediately asked my husband Justin to read the book, too. I let Justin know which techniques made the most sense to me and asked him to help me with them should they be needed. I saw his excitement grow as he read the book, and I could tell that he was on board for the ride.

I started talking to my baby all the time and forming what I felt was a true partnership. I would take walks and I would tell him (the baby) all about how I hoped our birth would go. By the eighth month, he already felt very low, and I had to accept the fact he might come before my Master's Thesis was complete (it was due a week before his due date), but I would remind him that his mom had some loose ends to tie up first and kindly encouraged him to hang tight.

During this pregnancy, I was determined to do whatever I could to prepare my body and mind for natural birth. I ate healthfully—lots of organic vegetables and protein. I drank lots of water. I stretched regularly and continued to take walks as my baby grew larger and larger. In addition to my regular multivitamin regimen, I took probiotics, extra calcium and magnesium to prevent leg cramps (something that plagued me in my previous pregnancy), extra folic acid, and added Raspberry Leaf supplements to my daily routine. I also drank Raspberry Leaf tea, hot and cold, to help condition my uterus, a recommendation of Sarah Najamy, another lovely midwife at the center. At night, I would listen to my HypnoBirthing meditation CD, a practice that helped both my daughter and me drift off to sleep peacefully together. Every day I continued to talk to my baby and envisioned the gentle, peaceful birth we both deserved.

Despite my best efforts to stay well, the mental and physical strain of my job was taking a toll on me. I could not ignore the fact that I started to slow down quite a bit in my last trimester. I was exhausted from my daily schedule—waking at 5:00 a.m., teaching on my feet all day long, and then digging deeper to find a second wind to play with my daughter until bedtime and try to be a good, involved mommy. The pressure on my abdomen was incredible. I started to develop varicose veins from all the standing necessary while teaching. Cathy Gallagher suggested I start wearing a bellyband to support the weight of my belly and support hose to help with the vein issue. Between the neoprene band hidden under my clothes and the confounding knee-highs, I was fit to burst. Poor Justin, what a turn I had taking from his blushing bride. I went out on maternity leave about one month before my due date to let my mind and body prepare for the birth, a decision I never second-guessed.

I am certain that the time off was instrumental in my having the kind of birth I desired. It afforded me the opportunity to keep my feet up much more than I could have otherwise, and gave me time to be mindful about my diet and exercise. That last month also gave me time to spend with Sofia and replenish our special bond before her brother arrived.

During this last month, I also read Ina May's first book, *Spiritual Midwifery*, which has more personal accounts of labor and delivery from ladies at The Farm in Tennessee, as well as a detailed guide and code of ethics for midwives to follow. The power of these narratives became profound to me. As I read each birth story, a feeling of being connected, part of a sisterhood, started to develop within me. My belief that birthing was a natural, normal process was strengthened. I also had the realization that a woman could make or break her own vision of birth—she just needed to wrap her head around that vision and hold tight … while also keeping her throat open and mooing like a cow (see chapter 19).

During my midwife visit the week before my son was due, I let Sarah Najamy know that I had been having fairly intense contractions at bedtime each night and felt like the baby's head was grinding lower and lower in my pelvic region. The contractions were not painful, just a lot of pressure. She asked me if I wanted her to check me for dilation. I explained that I needed two more days to complete and hand in my Thesis, and my boy and I had a pact not to go into labor until the paper was out of my hands. She smiled and said she would not check me then, for if I knew I was dilating, I might not be able to keep that pact, and she believed my mind power was working beautifully. This meeting helped to confirm my belief in myself and my love for midwives … I wonder how an OB/GYN would have reacted to the super mama mind power I believed I was harnessing.

Each night my boy and I would battle it out. Almost as soon as I would lie down, he would start moving and grooving. As crazy as it sounds, I swear I could feel the actual hair on the top of his head grinding against the bottom of my uterine wall. There was no position that would appease him. He would roll around and give me hell for at least two hours each night; all the while I would remind him of our deal. "Just three more days, Boy-O," I would say, "Only two days left until that paper will be done, *and then* we will meet." On a bright, sunny Friday in May, just five days before my due date, as I waddled around the campus of Western Connecticut State University obtaining the necessary faculty signatures for approval of my Thesis, I felt completely at peace with the world and full of accomplishment. I had finally completed my Master's degree, I had completed it on time, and my baby and I had kept our pact. I was now free to go into labor.

I had the wild notion that I would go into labor the minute I headed home from the campus. I felt exhausted from running around, and the baby felt like he was as low as he could be without falling right out. I made it home and finally could rest. The weekend passed without any signs of labor. How funny, I thought. My daughter had come ten days early. Now, only a few days away from my actual due date I started to wonder about this little man's agenda. Is he too comfortable in there?

The next day I took my daughter on a drive down the bumpiest roads I knew to try to get her to nap and shake this little guy down. Still nothing. I went for a walk down our country road, repeating "Mooooove Down ... Come out ... ," letting the words vibrate and move down my body to the baby, as I swung my arms forward and backwards. (It's a very quiet street, with no one around to enjoy this spectacle, save a few amused and confused squirrels). Still nothing. I decided to get as much rest as I could. He would make his move when he was ready. I waited for a sign.

I kept tabs on my appetite. The day I had gone into labor with Sofia I could hardly stand to eat anything. I figured I would let my appetite be a guide, but I continued to be ravenous, and actually began to worry that I might eat so much he would grow too large to come out easily. On Monday night Justin and I decided to give the nipple stimulation method that Ina May had recommended a try. After only about a minute, I immediately felt a contraction. Not like the pressurized contractions I had been experiencing for months, but a good old intense labor contraction! "Wow," I thought, "This really works!" I got scared and asked him to stop. Let's not force things, I told him, much to his displeasure (it was the first time I had let him near the girls in a good long time). I was impressed the method worked, but now wanted to let our boy make up his own mind.

The next morning I went for a pedicure. The woman who was polishing my toes asked politely, "When are you due?"

"In two days," I answered cheerily.

She grimaced. "You're not ready yet," she stated with an air of authority.

"Oh, yes I am!" I retorted. I was indeed ready ... It was my boy who was not quite ready to make his move.

That night I still had a hearty appetite at dinner. In bed I couldn't sleep and got up around 10:00 p.m., hungry again. Justin was still up watching Jon Stewart, so I joined him. As I wolfed down a big glob of lemon curd on toast, we joked that our boy was very comfy and would just come on his own time. I lay down on the couch and laughed through some of Jon Stewart's political nonsense and felt a strong contraction. It was 11:00 p.m. by this point and the contractions continued to come about every seven minutes. They were just strong enough that I was pretty sure I was experiencing the real thing, but I was in a bit of disbelief that they would continue.

When we went to bed, I let Justin know that the contractions were fairly regular and I thought it was really happening. I don't think he was really buying it, and he fell right to sleep. As Justin and Sofia slept beside me, I remembered my plan to stay open this time, to avoid clenching up. With each contraction I would stretch my head back and open my mouth as wide as it would go. If the contraction was particularly strong, I would also stick my tongue out as far as I could, Gene Simmons KISS Style. Simultaneously, I stretched my hands open, stretching my fingers as wide and straight as they could go. This routine gave me something other than the intensity of the contraction to focus on and the hours really flew by. I listened to the sounds of the night change as the tree frogs quieted and an owl began to hoot through the silence. I heard a train whistle blowing in the distance. As the hours passed, my excitement grew and I knew it wouldn't be long before I met our little man.

At four o'clock I had to get out of bed. I was having a hard time lying down at this point, and I suddenly felt that I would have an accident of the seriously messy kind if I didn't get to the bathroom quick. I decided to go out to our kitchen and let Justin and Sofia sleep. I was right about the bathroom … three flushes later, I was quite sure I was cleaned out. Another good sign, I thought. My body was getting ready for the birth.

The contractions were getting very strong and I found squatting to be helpful. I held onto my kitchen counter top and squatted down during each surge, continuing to throw my head back and stick my tongue out. I was glad no one was watching me. I felt free to be as weird as I needed to be. I also found it helpful to make a deep AAAAAAAA sound as my tongue was out. Sort of an extended version of what a doctor asks you to do when he or she puts the tongue depressor in your mouth. The contractions were about four to five minutes apart at this point, but I had a goal to wait until the sun came up to alert Justin, the midwife, and my husband's sister who was going to look after Sofia during the birth. To wait out the two hours, I made myself a cup of mint tea and popped *Bridget Jones's Diary* in the DVD player.

I sat on the couch with our dog, Clarice, sipping the hot tea, and enjoying the calming stability of Colin Firth's dreamy eyes in between contractions. I started a new routine during this phase of contractions. I opened my hands up wide and rode the wave of each contraction. I would set my gaze at the spot where the wall met the ceiling and let my eyes and head follow the beam that crossed over the ceiling over my head slowly up until my neck was fully extended back and my tongue was jutting out all the way. As the contraction diminished, I would follow the beam back down as slowly as I had followed it up. This, again, was a transfer of focus, which really helped to take my mind off the intensity. Clarice looked up at me from time to time, as she kept my feet warm. It was during this time that I also started hearing Cat Steven's song playing in my head, "I can't keep it in … can't keep it in, I gotta let it out!"—a song one of Ina May's ladies wrote about as a stress reliever during her labor. Those cheery words jangled around in my mind for about an hour and kept me moving forward with a happy kind of excitement until Colin Firth and Hugh Grant hurled themselves through a plate glass window in foolish leading movie brawl style, and "It's Raining Men" drowned Cat out. Hallelujah! I was almost there!

My labor with Sofia had taken 32 hours from the first contraction to her birth, but I was sure this one was going to be much different and had convinced myself that this baby would be born around 10:00 or 11:00 a.m. When the movie ended and the first hints of daylight appeared, I moved back into the bedroom and climbed into bed. Justin opened his eyes and I told him that it was really happening. He watched me as I did my Gene Simmons impersonations, and I told him it was time to call his sister. He asked me if he should drive Sofia down.

"No … they need to come get her … you are going to need to take me to have a baby."

He was surprised that I was as far along as I claimed to be, but got out of bed and made the call, as a sleepy Sofia started to wake. I sat down on the chaise in our bedroom as Justin got Sofia dressed, and I explained to her that she would be meeting her brother today. It was important to me that she know that this was it … mommy was going to have the baby soon, but she didn't need to worry or have any fear, so I just breathed calmly and smiled. I didn't want her to think labor was scary. She looked at me with so much tenderness and understanding in her eyes. I was extremely touched that our two-year-old seemed to be sensing the gravity of the moment, and she came over and kissed my belly, looked up into my eyes, and told me she loved me. I continued to breathe slowly through the contractions as we shared this time together.

I asked Justin to call the answering service for our midwife and explain that I was in labor. We actually had an appointment to meet with the Cathy Parisi scheduled for that morning at 9:30 a.m., so I asked him to mention that when he called in. I really wanted Cathy Parisi to be the midwife attending my second birth since I felt she did such a fantastic job making tough calls and sticking up for us during my first experience.

Our brother-in-law, Tom, arrived quickly to take Sofia to his house, and I immediately started running warm water into the bath tub. I just needed to be in there. Justin returned to me as I climbed into the tub and started splashing the warm water over my big belly. He informed me that he called the birth center and left the message that I was in labor, and we would be in for our 9:30 appointment.

"What?" I shook my head, "I'm having this baby NOW … no, no, no … you misunderstood me … Call back … We are going in NOW!"

"Then why are you in the tub?"

Now, to be fair to Justin, I was playing it super cool in front of Sofia. I had not clearly explained what I was feeling or even that my contractions were about three minutes apart. So, the poor guy was shocked when I showed these first signs of unrest. I calmed myself down.

"It's okay. It's okay. Cathy will call back soon to confirm she got the message and we can tell her then. Anyhow, my water hasn't broken yet, so we probably have a little time."

Now by this point, some of you readers may be shaking your own heads, wondering why on Earth I was still at home at all, let alone in a bath tub. I can't say I was right to wait that long, but I was just doing what made sense to me. I was fairly certain that my baby was not in any kind of distress. Unlike Sofia, who I could not feel move at all during that labor, who unbeknownst to me until hours into it had her cord wrapped around her neck, this little bugger was up to his usual tricks—shifting around, grinding his head lower, and kicking me. I took this as a sign that he was working with me, not against me. I felt like I was in as much control of the situation as possible, and I honestly felt everything would turn out well.

Just as I began to feel like I was finding a little comfort in the warm water … . POW!!!!!! An unexpected burst … an explosion. I almost expected to look down and see a little fist sticking out of me. I'm pretty sure I actually heard a POP.

"My water just broke! Do you see anything?"

"A little blood."

The phone rang. It was Cathy Parisi.

"Her water just broke Cathy … She's in the tub … How far along are your contractions, babe?

"Two minutes!"

My stomach began to shudder uncontrollably and I had to crunch myself forward to get a handle on the sensation. The thought flashed across my mind that I might be having this baby in the tub momentarily. Justin stood over me and watched as the labor took on a new dimension. It was intense. I put my hand over my crotch and decided I did not want the local volunteer firefighters to be hovering over me as I lay naked in my tub with my newborn in my arms. No, I would make it to the birth center. I was determined.

When my belly stopped shuddering, Justin very calmly brought me a towel.

"Cathy says I need to get you to the birth center now. Let's do this, mama!"

Justin helped me get up and out of the tub and held me through the next contraction. I found holding him tightly and asking him to hug me harder helped ease the intensity. He helped me get dressed quickly—into my giant pregnancy undies—no time for a bra. I had two more contractions on the way out to the car and he held me tight through both of them. I waddled into the car and full speed ahead into the most psychedelic trip of my life.

Now, I have never tried psychedelic drugs, and half rolled my eyes during the Ina May birth stories that kept describing the births as "psychedelic" and making the ladies feel "high." Whatever, I thought. Well, as we drove the 40 minutes to the birth center I swear I experienced a completely altered state. I had my eyes closed for most of it as we raced through country back roads around soft turns. The few times I opened my eyes the landscapes we passed looked like long flowing green lines. I was also seriously sweating and needed to have the window down to cool me as we raced. I couldn't sit down and rode with my body rigid as a plank, feet on the front of the foot compartment, one hand holding tightly to the sunroof, the other firmly between my legs. With each contraction, my belly shook and I needed to push to ease the feeling. So I pushed against my hand, which was holding our boy in, and I breathed. Short breaths when that felt right, long ones when that felt right. I opened my eyes when we were close and told Justin what a great job he was doing getting me there fast. I knew how stressed he must be as the driver and really wanted to help him stay calm, too.

We called the birth center from my cell phone en route to ask that they fill up the birthing tub. They were already doing it, they assured me.

We pulled up. It was a beautiful sunny day. Bright, crisp blue sky. Cathy was waiting at the door for me.

"How we doing, mama?"

"I'm holding him in, Cathy."

"I can see that," she smiled.

Justin and Cathy helped me to the birthing room and through to the bathroom where the tub was waiting for me. Cathy wanted to check the baby's heart rate before I got into the tub, and she waited until another contraction passed to do so.

"Sounds good! Get in the tub. I will check your dilation once you get in."

They helped me into the tub and Ahhhhhhhhhhh … the pain drifted away instantaneously. No joke … pain gone.

"His head is right there. You can push when you're ready."

I love Cathy Parisi. She keeps a scene so cool and natural.

"What should I do?"

"Just do what feels right. Push when you feel a contraction."

On the next contraction, I pushed, but didn't feel like the baby budged. I grabbed hold of my upper thighs close to the groin, first from the front, then from the back, just trying to get a good grip on myself, so I could use my body to create greater resistance to push this baby out. I got a handle on the feeling and pushed really hard into my bottom to move him on down. I started to feel his head coming through and a slight stinging sensation as he made his way out. The stinging was not overwhelming, and there was no other pain. Cathy and Justin were really great. Cathy kept saying, "You're doing it, you're doing it!" and helping me up when my head started to slip below the water. I felt a little frustrated when my baby's head started coming out, then would retreat back in, but Cathy reassured me that this was exactly what was supposed to happen to allow me to stretch out as needed. Whenever I looked up at Justin, I could tell I was doing a good job because he was smiling from ear to ear. As our son's head was coming out, Cathy would play around with the baby's hair and waft the water around towards me to sooth the area.

"He's got a lot of hair," she confirmed.

The whole experience felt exceptionally surreal. I was in the warm tub and the whole room seemed to envelope me in a warm, loving glow. The shades were drawn and lights were dimmed. It actually struck me at the time as being a very romantic setting. It didn't feel like I was pushing for very long when I felt the head come out completely. I looked down to see and gave another great push and out came the rest of our boy into the water.

"Pick him up, Mama," Cathy said.

And so I did. I reached down and lifted our son to my chest and took him in. He looked great. Cathy cleared his airways as I held him in the tub. She checked his heart. All was perfect. Justin knelt down and cut the cord. Our son was here—healthy and noticeably strong. Justin took Emmett into his arms as Cathy and the nurse, Heather, helped me out of the tub.

As I dried off, Justin walked around the room with our son in his arms. I climbed up on the bed and began to nurse Emmett as Cathy stitched up a little tear. Emmett latched right on and made me feel like a breastfeeding phenom. He was so calm. He didn't fuss at all while the nurse measured and weighed him, just looked around at everyone and seemed generally pleased.

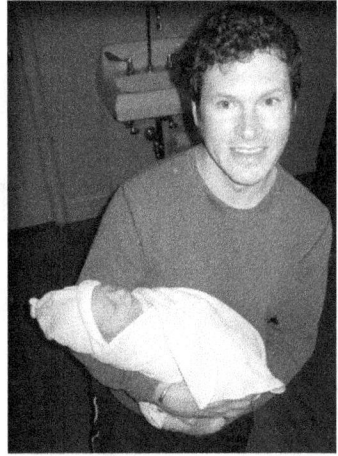

Justin holding Emmett for his first picture

Our nurse was there to help us with anything we needed when Cathy had to run across the street to attend a woman who was birthing at the hospital. We spent the morning resting in the totally peaceful birthing suite, my baby in my arms, nursing, smiling, sleeping. A warm breeze blew in through the open window. We listened to our own music, ate, and relaxed happily. It really was ideal.

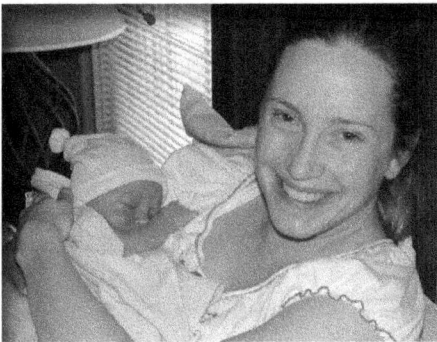

Natasha and Emmett shortly after the birth

The first day that Emmett joined us out in the big, wide world was truly divine. After about an hour of resting on the bed, I decided I needed to shower. Heather helped me to the bathroom. As I entered the bathroom I realized it looked much different now than my memory of it during the birth. The birthing tub, in fact, was about 45 degrees turned from where I remembered it to be and there were no candles lit, or any candles at all, for that matter. I realized in that moment that I really had been in an altered state during the birth, and because of my calmness and the positive outlook I had towards the entire experience, I saw that bathroom to be much more beautiful than it ever was. But that's pretty wild, isn't it? Ina May's ladies were right ... birth is a far out, psychedelic mind trip.

Justin's sister, Jenny, brought our daughter Sofia to the Birth Center around noon to meet her brother. It was a very happy time. Justin retold the tale of his wife's quick labor and "rock star" birthing to our visitors and everyone he called. As I rested on the bed with my healthy son in my arms, I felt incredible. Tired, yes, but incredible. I felt like I had accomplished exactly

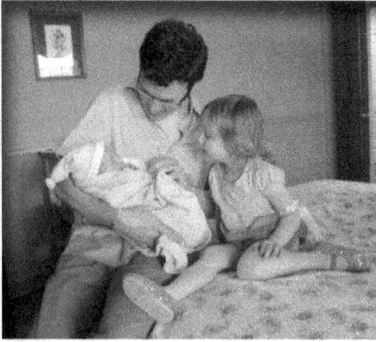

Sofia meeting her brother

what I had set out to. I had labored at home. I had remained calm. I used the techniques that felt right to remain unclenched. I didn't feel like I needed any medications, and I didn't end up in the hospital. I made it to the Birth Center on time, and I popped that baby out in what felt like lightning speed in retrospect. As I reviewed the timetable of my labor and delivery, I felt proud.

11:00 p.m.: First contractions

7:15 a.m.: Water broke at home

8:15 a.m.: Arrived at the birth center

8:30 a.m.: Emmett Joseph Wildwood was born in the tub, 7 pounds 8 ounces, 19 inches long.

What a high! The more I thought about the whole experience the more empowered I became. When I set out to have this type of a birth, I thought it would be good for me—good for my soul, something I needed to prove to myself, something I wanted to do for my son. I never realized how wonderful it would make me feel until the little guy was in my arms, and I was sure it was the best I could have done for both him and me.

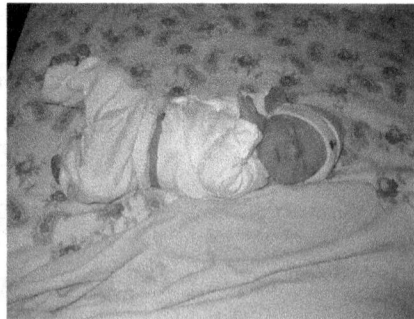

Emmett ready to go home

After our relatives left, Justin went out to the living room to let Emmett and I take our first nap together. Having been up all night in labor, I was good and ready to sleep and fell out quickly. When I woke up a little later, I felt refreshed and ready to go. I slowly got myself and the baby dressed, and we packed our bags. Cathy came back from the hospital just in time to give us all hugs and wish us well. We were on our way back home at 4:00 p.m. The sun was shining and we all felt great.

I took it easy for the week after the birth. Justin stayed home from work to be with Sofia, so I could get as much rest as possible. I took Motrin to ease the soreness, but otherwise I felt really good. I was happy not to have the back pain I had from the epidural or the uncomfortable peeing sensation from the catheter after my first birth. I could walk around the house with minimal discomfort and felt ready to tackle the new responsibilities of being a mother of two.

Emmett showed every sign of being healthy and strong. He was exceptionally alert, even from the first day, making good eye contact with everyone. He could hold his head up very early and had remarkable strength for a newborn during his first week. We were so pleased. I know that every baby is different, but I believe the choices I made while I was pregnant and during labor and delivery had a lot to do with the outcome, our totally magnificent boy.

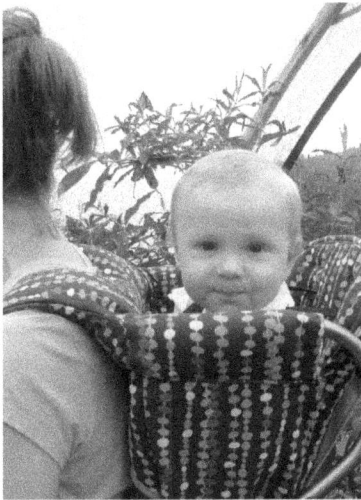

Emmett at one year

Mine is not one of those stories claiming that labor and birth are pain free or a breeze, but I think it does help to show the importance of the experience. Women need to take back their birthing rights, believe in themselves, and embrace the awesome transformative power of natural childbirth, an experience that is immeasurably meaningful and profoundly beneficial, not only for baby and mama, but for society as a whole.

3

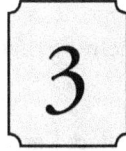

Aster's Birth Story: Why I chose Hypnobabies

By Cassie Friesen

When I first became pregnant, I was terrified of the actual birthing part. I had watched Hollywood's version of birth for far too long, and the images of sheer terror in these mothers had imprinted itself in my brain. I had the impression that you lose all control due to the excruciating amount of pain, but it would be completely worth it because it's the most amazing day of your life and the pain is such a small price to pay ... blah, blah, blah. Well, I wasn't thrilled at my options. On the one hand, I really wanted to experience a natural birth because of the uniqueness of an experience that only women can share in, but I really wasn't interested in the amount of pain I perceived was inevitable. The other option was to receive an epidural to help numb the pain, but be unable to be fully in tune with my body and experience the process. It was at that point that I began looking into my childbirth options.

I remembered when my best friend had her baby at a birthing center the year before that I had seen a brochure for HypnoBirthing. It sounded very strange to me and, of course, I said, "I'd be willing to try anything if it meant I could avoid the pain!" It was an ignorant statement said with images of being completely unconscious and under someone else's 'control' flickering through my brain. Well, by the time I was a couple months pregnant and researching different childbirth preparation courses, I decided to look into different types of hypnosis for childbirth. I came across Hypnobabies and decided to read some of the birth stories and watch the birth videos on YouTube. I tried desperately to search for negative reviews in Google's search engine. I only came across positive birth experiences, and the women seemed so happy with the program. Many of them even had pain-free births! I decided to put all of my effort into it, and my husband, Peter, was happy to be my birth partner and become very involved as well. I didn't want to participate in something that sounded so far-fetched without giving it my all.

There weren't any local classes offered at the time, so I ordered the home study program. I have the type of personality that I knew would work well to invest a lot of time and energy into this program on my own; I'm definitely not a procrastinator and started the program early at 26 weeks. What I immediately realized was that Hypnobabies is all about listening to your body, relaxing, embracing change, releasing fears, and enjoying every moment of your pregnancy for what it is. There's a *Joyful Pregnancy Affirmations* CD that I listened to every day, and it made me feel so powerful and grateful to be experiencing what I was going through. It also helped me love all the changes that were occurring in my body. There are several other CDs that you cycle through and practice, like *Your Special Place Imagery and Relaxation, Easy, Comfortable Childbirth*, and *Fear Clearing Session*. The most important part of Hypnobabies was to practice the different "switches," like a mental light switch. When you "switch off," you go completely limp and relax every muscle in your body, and think about moving mental anesthesia to different parts of your body that need it. When you are in "center switch," you are still deeply relaxed, but are able to move around, talk, and function as normal. In the "on position," you are fully conscious and in your normal state. They urge you to practice these switches, so when your birthing time comes, you can fully participate in them without thinking about it.

Hypnobabies uses different vocabulary than your typical childbirth course because they are trying to change the way your mind perceives childbirth. Instead of laboring, you're birthing; contractions are pressure waves; there is no false labor, only practice birthing/pressure waves; due dates are guess dates because the baby picks his/her birthday... I thought that it seemed a little corny and, at first, I especially hated asking people to use this terminology around me if they would be speaking of birthing for any length of time. Hypnobabies has you create a bubble of peace and that really put me over the edge. The idea behind the peace bubble was that everything good and supportive of me and my birthing choices were in the bubble with me, and anything negative bounced off the bubble. I was surprised at how helpful it was once I got past how absolutely bizarre it sounded. And one of the most important messages Hypnobabies reiterates is that whatever birth experience you have is the perfect one for you. So it's great to plan and visualize what your birth will be like, but if you end up needing a C-section or an emergency transfer, that may very well be what was perfect for you; it's important to be flexible when there are so many variables at work.

Let's fast forward to my birthing time. On July 6th I was completely unaware that my early pressure waves had begun. The ones I experienced were stronger and a little different than Braxton Hicks had been, but I still felt like I was having Braxton Hicks, in addition to these new ones. I didn't think anything of it and would simply adjust the way I sat or breathe a little more deeply when they occurred. I experienced them periodically throughout the day and while we were out at dinner with my husband, my in-laws, and their friends. That evening around 12:00 p.m. I told my husband that I thought the pressure waves might actually be the real thing, but I wasn't sure because I was actually enjoying how powerful and strong they were. We went to bed excited, but with little expectation.

Almost immediately I noticed them getting stronger and occurring with more regularity, but I was so sleepy and felt like I was in a dreamlike state that I still didn't think anything of it. When each one occurred, I would close my eyes, breathe deeply, and relax my body. I visualized a deep, undulating sound as I gently body surfed up and down over continuous waves. (I assume that I visualized this because I had called contractions 'pressure waves' for so long). Each wave grew stronger, and then gradually weaker, and they only lasted about a minute each it seemed. After each one I would smile, just like the program had taught me to, because they were bringing my baby that much closer to meeting me. That's when I finally remembered that Braxton Hicks go away when you lay down and true pressure waves do not. I didn't see the point in waking Peter up, so I continued to experience them consistently until 2:30ish in the morning. The only pregnancy symptom I had was severe heartburn throughout the entire pregnancy, and it struck at that time. I didn't want to get up and find my Tums, so I woke Peter up and calmly explained that I was having real pressure waves, but, unfortunately, my heartburn was acting up and asked him to please get my Tums. He asked me a few questions. As I was explaining how I was feeling and what the pressure waves were like, I felt a 'pop' at 2:47 a.m. and said, "Well, I think my water just broke. I'll go use the restroom and check it out while you get the Tums." Sure enough, I was leaking a little bit. I threw a pad on and laid back down to continue my pressure waves.

I threw up the first time about 3:30 a.m., but wasn't too concerned. I had an upset stomach and was using the restroom quite often after the waves, but I vaguely remembered that being common when your birthing time is imminent. Then I noticed that while deep breathing through pressure waves I felt like I was going to throw up. Sure enough, I did, and it seemed like I threw up with every pressure wave that was exceptionally strong. I was slightly discouraged because all of my practicing had been built upon deep breathing, and it seemed as though I wouldn't be able to do that. But I quickly figured out a way to breathe a bit more shallowly, and I didn't seem to throw up quite as often as I felt my body wanted to. Peter timed the waves until 4:18 a.m.; some were three minutes apart, others nine minutes, so we decided to get some sleep. We fell asleep for about four hours, and I woke up long enough to breathe through the waves before I fell back to sleep. I listened to the 'Birth-Day Affirmations' while I was sleeping. Throughout the rest of the morning I listened to different CDs, depending on which one I felt would be the most useful at that moment in time.

I continued to have pressure waves all morning. Peter kept me well hydrated and occasionally timed them. When the pressure waves were getting more frequent, Peter drew me a warm bath and I hung out in there for a long time while I listened to my CDs and focused on relaxing and breathing deeply. In between checking on me and timing the pressure waves, Peter gathered our last minute supplies for the birth bag, so it would be ready to go by the time I was. While I was in the tub, the pressure waves became much stronger. I had him stay to support my body, so I could be completely limp during them.

Eventually, I decided I'd be more comfortable lying back down in bed, so I headed over there and continued to have much stronger pressure waves. At this point, I began low moaning for the duration of each pressure wave. I'm not sure when it was that I informed Peter the moaning was not from pain—I was doing what my body was telling me to do and it felt good to make these noises. I think that helped him relax. I began feeling 'pushy' around 11:30 a.m. and had two or three involuntary pushes. I asked Peter to call the midwife because I thought it might be time to go in. The pressure waves were coming three to five minutes apart, and because they had been so strong for a while, the midwife told Peter to have us head down. He got the car packed and brought several pillows, so I could prop myself up comfortably during the ride. This allowed me to go limp during the pressure waves while in the car. We left around 12:15 p.m. Peter did a wonderful job driving calmly (even if he wasn't feeling very calm!), while I kept my eyes shut and continued to listen to my CDs with my headphones on and moan deeply with the pressure waves. On the drive I threw up into the wastebasket that Peter had so wisely packed. Peter has since told me that some of the waves came two minutes apart, which made him nervous that we would be birthing roadside. I guess I had a break for about seven minutes, and he hoped we'd have enough time to get to the birth center. The birth center is about 40 minutes away and we arrived just after 1:00 p.m. I waited until one pressure wave had passed before I got out of the car. I made it to the bench outside of the birthing center and asked Peter if we could sit down for another pressure wave before we headed upstairs. When we got upstairs I laid down in the room I knew I would be birthing in, while Peter went to find someone, since everyone was eating out on the balcony.

Laura, a midwife in training, came in to do a vaginal exam. I asked her how long those take and she said about a minute. I told her to wait since another pressure wave was coming on. When I 'came up' from it, I told her she should probably get in there quick before the baby came. She laughed and apparently thought I was at about 4 cm since I was in such a good mood and joking around with her. While she was doing the exam, she said, "I can't find the cervix." I naively asked, "Where did it go?" She said, "That means you're at 10 cm … ." I responded, "Well, that's good, right?" She asked the midwife, Tracy, if she could check to make sure she wasn't wrong, and I told them that didn't seem necessary because I didn't have trouble believing I was that close. On a side note, Hypnobabies encourages you to have a birthing dayproject for your early birthing time. They suggest making a sweet treat for whoever will be attending the birth. I apologized to everyone for not making cookies or brownies for them since I hadn't realized I was in my birthing time and that just made them laugh. Poor Peter wanted five minutes to eat some of his protein bar, go to the bathroom, and get his swim trunks on since we were going to be in the water tub, and I told him, "Baby's waiting on you!" I had another pressure wave and the midwives rubbed my back while he was gone.

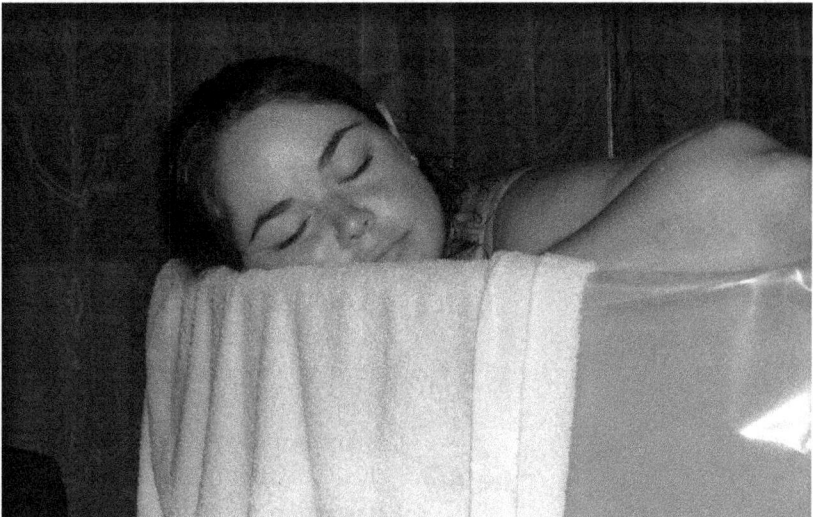

Cassie relaxing in the birthing tub

When he got back, we both got in the water tub, and he massaged my lower back during all of my pressure waves. In between we were joking around with the midwives and one another. I was still feeling great and totally relaxed between them.

These pressure waves felt so much more powerful that my moaning almost felt like a low roar, bellowing up from somewhere so deep inside me that I don't think I could ever imitate it again without being in my actual birthing time. I've learned that those noises are fairly common with natural births, especially those using hypnosis, and have been compared to a weight lifter or martial artist. You don't see a weight lifter or martial artist quietly lifting heavy weights or breaking through bricks without noise—there is an enormous amount of energy behind the groans you hear them make. It felt the same for me, very powerful.

Hypnobabies had prepared me for the 'breathing baby out' phase as a two steps forward, one step back process. That's exactly what it felt like—it was a great practice in patience. The midwives put a mirror below where the labia was parting, so I could see her hair floating in the water and see where to touch the top of her head—her hair was so soft! The amount of hair confirmed a reason for the severe heartburn. I 'pushed'/breathed baby out for an hour and a half or two hours, and the only complaint I had during it was that my heartburn was making me throw up a little in my mouth during my low moaning. Tracy got a bowl and told me I could spit into it, but the first time I did, it bounced back and hit me in the face. I joked, "Well, that didn't work out so well." Throughout the whole time we were in the tub I'd ask Peter if he was having fun or how he was doing, and his response was always some version of, "Time of my life, baby." When he asked me how I was doing, my responses varied from how much fun I was having, that the baby and I made a great team, or what a good birth partner Peter was.

During the birthing stage and anytime the pressure waves were more

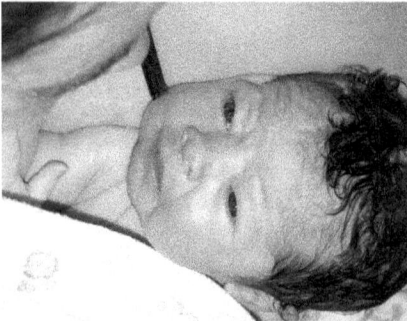

Baby Aster just born

intense, I used the "peace" cue. This meant I exhaled deeply as I said, "Peeeeeaaaace" and imagined breathing mental anesthesia to wherever I felt my body needed it. It was probably the most useful cue that I employed and really allowed me to focus on something. I had a little trouble maintaining relaxation once she was crowning. Peter repeated some of the relaxation cues, which helped me immensely. I was leaned forward over the tub's edge and Peter was behind me the whole time. As she was coming out, Pete was updating me on how far she was and I heard him say, "She has your nose! Thank God!" He caught her and the midwives helped pull her up between my legs and laid her in my arms. Pete was crying and I was just staring at her in awe when Pete asked, "Is it a boy or girl?" Laura told us she hadn't seen yet, and then checked- it was a girl! We said, "Hello, Aster!" After nine months of not knowing who this little person was that grew inside me, it was amazing to finally meet her.

The news of Aster's birth spread like wildfire throughout the birth center. At our checkups since the birth, we've been told by midwives, even those not in attendance, how impressed they were. One midwife told me I birthed like a second time mom, only better. Another said that she knew I would do well since I had practiced religiously. The ones who attended the birth laughed about how silly Peter and I were during my birthing time, and especially how I apologized for not baking them cookies. Laura informed us that on their student blog everyone was talking about different births they'd witnessed, and she told them, "I got to see a pain-free birth; it was incredible!"

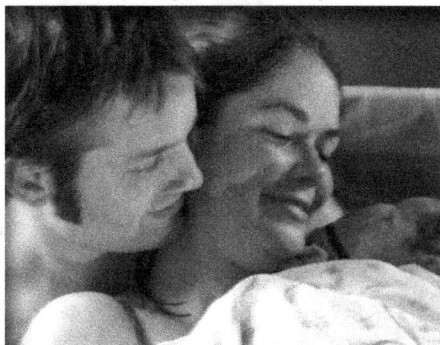

Peter and Cassie admiring baby Aster

You won't ever hear me say that Hypnobabies is the only or best childbirth course. I feel like this is one of those decisions that is very personal, and each woman needs to pick what will make her the most comfortable. This was perfect for me. But the only reason it worked as well as it did was because I practiced. I'm sure the same would be true for other childbirth courses if they were practiced as much. A runner doesn't show up at a marathon never having run a day in his/her life and expect to be successful. Birthing is a tremendous event and requires a lot of time and energy. I was pleased that my training paid off. Mostly, what I learned from this experience is that birth doesn't have to be an out-of-control event, and I was surprised to find it could actually be comfortable, enjoyable, and even fun.

4

The Journey to Meeting my Sweet Baby Evelynn

By Rachel Sobolewski

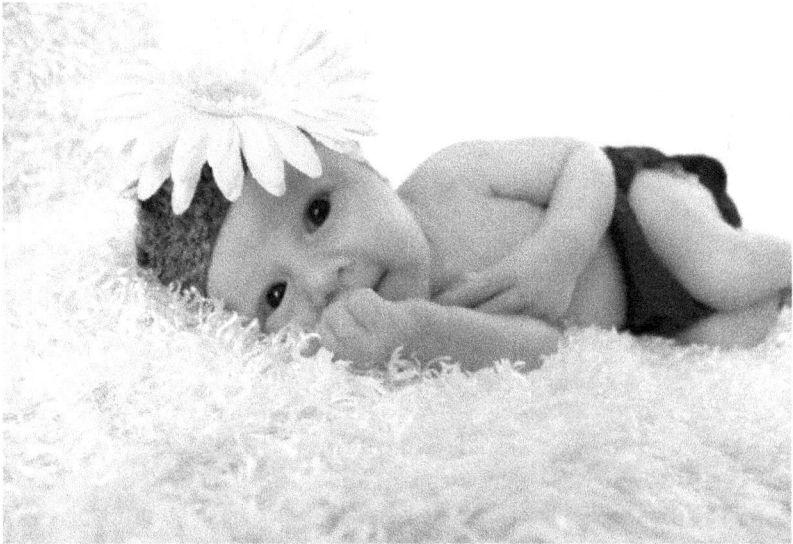

Baby Evvie at two weeks old

I believe that stories have the power to change lives, inspire others, and build a sense of commonality amongst all human kind. One of the most universal experiences across cultures is the experience of childbirth. It is also one of the most amazing, transformative, and powerful experiences I believe I will ever have. Therefore, I think that the story of a birth, as honest as it may be, needs to be shared...at least with those who choose to read it.

My birth story technically started about a year and a half ago, when I discovered a documentary called *The Business of Being Born* on Netflix. My husband Steve was in the living room playing one of his shooting games on the Xbox. I was helplessly bored, so I sat down with our laptop and decided to watch the movie. I have been fascinated with babies and childbirth my entire life and have even been teased by my friends for watching every episode of TLC's "A Baby Story;" some more than once. There was just something so miraculous about a new life, and people's birth stories fascinated me to no end. This night was different, however. After watching the documentary, I was so thrown off by the idea that birth could be different than the classic panic-filled, starch white, hooked-up-to-a-million-things-at-once hospital room that I couldn't sleep. And Steve, who was not nearly as interested in childbirth as I was, grew disinterested in hearing facts about childbirth in the United States.

My passion for natural childbirth started to grow as I read more and more information. Facts were coming in from everywhere I could get them, and my friends were probably learning more about birth than they cared to. I learned that the United States has terrible statistics for mother and child health, and we are one of the only countries that use hospitals for birth. Our C-section rate is over three times what the World Health Organization (a result of needless interventions) says is safe.... and the list goes on and on. But the most important thing I learned was the idea that natural birth is healthier and easier on the mom and baby, and the countries that choose natural home births for low risk pregnancies were at the top of the list for health and success. For the first time, I was faced with the idea that my body was made to birth, and that if other women could do it every day all over the world, I could do it, too. I was sold. I even considered switching my education mid-master's program to become a midwife, but let's face it, I didn't want to have to take biochemistry.

There was only one problem...I had never given birth. In April of 2009, however, my prospects would change. Steve and I, after 8 months of marriage, discovered we were pregnant and due in January (ready or not!), January 25th to be exact. The first step I took when I found out I was pregnant was contacting Morning Star birth center in St. Louis Park, MN. I wanted to avoid the hospital system completely. I had come across their website in all of my natural birth research, which ended up coming in handy! At four weeks gestation, we went in for a site visit, and Steve and I decided this was the place our little one would enter the world.

Fast forward nine months of cravings, tears, and heartburn to January 24th, 2011. I was feeling pretty good and confident about the impending labor on the morning of January 24th when I started to get some annoying cramps around 7:30 a.m. I tried to calm my excitement by assuring myself it was Braxton-Hicks. I spent the entire day telling myself, "I'm not going to call until it's real." The entire day I kept cramping up, but nothing too uncomfortable, so I just kept going on with my everyday life...I even went to work (I work in a retail makeup store) that night with the idea that I didn't want to be embarrassed if it was false labor. After all, most first babies are born almost two weeks late!

However, as I spent more time at work, I realized that it probably was not false labor I was experiencing and called Steve to come pick me up. We drove to the grocery store to pick up food for the labor and after the birth, and I grew increasingly anxious with the idea that this was "it." So much for my complete confidence, I was getting nervous!

I wasn't really sure how to manage the pain at that time. I think my anxiety about the upcoming experience was getting to me and keeping me from relaxing and just going with the contractions. When a contraction would come, I would rock back and forth and cry, because I was getting nervous that this was finally it!

I called my two friends that would attend the birth with me to come over, because I was "ready" to go. My contractions were two minutes apart for over an hour, and I was sure that if it hurt this bad, I must be having this baby tonight. However, when I called Catherine, my midwife, she told me that it sounded like this was my day, but not quite my time. I was freaking out. How could it not be time? I was in so much pain and my contractions were two minutes apart, what else needed to happen first? I was about to find out.

We left about an hour after the phone call because I was sure there had to be some sort of mistake. After an hour in the car, we reached the birth center. I managed my pain in the car by remembering to breathe through the contractions and by focusing on timing, knowing they would be over in about a minute. When we went inside to get checked, my blood pressure was quite high (anyone who knows me well would not be surprised about that) and I was almost in a panic. (Again, I wondered where did all of my confidence go?) Then Catherine checked me. She said I was a "tight 3" ... which was the nice way of saying I was not even dilated to three yet. I had a long way to go.

Catherine suggested I get into the Jacuzzi tub and try to relax a bit. Within a minute of being in the water, the pain subsided a bit and my blood pressure came down. I was able to relax my breathing and refocus on what needed to be done—my little girl needed to greet the world. The labor was intense throughout the entire night. I found myself getting upset when new techniques were suggested to me. Didn't anyone understand that I was in PAIN?! Why would I want to move around or try uncomfortable positions? I could tell my attitude was becoming pretty irrational... I remember saying out loud, "I wish I was anyone else in this room but me right now!" I was losing it...no amount of planning could have prepared me for that type of pain. Looking back on the experience, I now realize that these positions were what made the labor progress...there is so much wisdom in methods like walking the stairs and swinging your hips and doing lunges ... methods that are now thrown out the window by modern medicine. Though I didn't want to rock my hips through a contraction, the motion really helped to drop baby Evelynn down into my pelvis, and I cannot imagine laboring without the relief of a Jacuzzi tub! Although these methods are different than a typical birth in America, they really helped!

By around noon on the 25th, I was becoming pretty exhausted. Catherine checked me (at my insistence) and said I was about an 8. An 8?!? How could it be? It was then that she said that part of my cervix was swollen, which might have been why I wasn't dilating. My midwife said that an option was for me to get out of the water (I had planned to do a water birth), so she could stretch my cervix by hand, over the baby. I jumped at the opportunity. I was so ready to be done. Almost instantly (at least it felt like it to me), my water broke and I was ready to push. After pushing on my back for a while, I knew it was not working for me. So I decided to stand up, something I had never considered beforehand while I was planning my quiet, calm, water birth. I was screaming and moaning. I was loud and complaining. This was not how I had pictured myself! Holding on to Steve, I pushed as hard as I could. I remember Paula (another midwife at Morningstar) coming in, just in time, and telling me that I was beautiful. That is one of the few memories I have. I felt like giving up when she was almost out, until Catherine said, "Rachel, a few more pushes and you will be holding your baby!" This gave me the strength to get her out. At 2:30 pm, after an hour and a half of pushing, Evelynn Rebecca was born, right on her due date! Turns out she's a planner, just like her Mommy!

I laid back on the bed and the 7 pound, 8.5 ounce little girl was laid across my chest. Evelynn was born with her hand on her head, which could have caused the delay ... what a little stinker! (To this day she has to sleep with that little hand by her face!) She was having trouble breathing at first, but everyone was so calm that I didn't have time to panic. Her little eyes were open and looking around at everything, and I was in a complete state of shock. Evelynn was still getting oxygen through the cord, which the midwives left attached until it was done pulsing, a procedure which allows all of the baby's blood supply to pump back into the baby. The midwives were sucking the junk from Evelynn's mouth and nose and giving her oxygen to help her breathe. All the while, she was on my chest with me, right where I could see her and know that she was all right. Soon enough, she was breathing fine and she tested out her lungs with a cute little cry. I was so out of it from being up and in labor for two days it took me a while to cry, but I did. She was so beautiful and perfect!

We were able to take an herbal bath as a family, which was relaxing and wonderful after the labor! All the while, Evvie was alert and awake, not bogged down by any drugs. She was too cute to handle! Steve and I talked about the birth and how happy we were with our new little girl, and, for the first time in 30 hours, we relaxed. When we were ready, about five hours later, we were able to go home and crawl into our own bed with our new baby girl. She even slept most of the night; turns out she was exhausted, too!

As I write this story, six weeks after the birth, I still cannot believe I was able to do it. I do not seem like an obvious candidate for a natural birth. I am a young mom, and to be honest, I'm really not that mature. I head straight for conventional medicine when I am sick, and I am a bit of a complainer when it comes to pain. Even so, I knew birth was different. I am so thankful for the experience I had at Morning Star. It took me a while to be okay with the fact that I was not calm and stoic like I had envisioned myself being. I had to come to terms with the fact that when Evvie was born it took me a while to really connect with her because I was exhausted and shocked. Every other natural birth story I had read seemed like the women were so put together the entire time and completely restored after the birth, and that wasn't me. But that's ok. That is why I found it important to share my story. Even though I had researched and asked a million questions, there was no way to fully prepare for labor and birth. However, it worked. My body knew what to do and had the wisdom to bring Evelynn into this world safely. If I could do it, anyone can do it!

My birth was an amazing experience and the most difficult thing I have ever done, yet I wouldn't change a thing. Steve was the most supportive birth partner I could have ever asked for, and now a huge advocate for natural childbirth! Everyone attending the birth made it an encouraging and positive experience. Having supportive friends who believed in the natural process really helped me stay focused and feel supported. One friend even gave up most of her own birthday (Evvie was born the same day!) to be with me during the birth. I never knew that I could form such amazing relationships with the midwives and the assistants, but we were actually sad leaving our six-week appointment, knowing that it was the end (or the beginning!) of a life-changing journey.

At the end of the experience of pregnancy and birth, I only have one hope. I hope Evelynn knows forever how much her mommy loves her, that I did my best to do what was best for her, and that I would do it again a million times over just to have her in my life!

5

The Birth of Elijah Jayden Tendler

By Krista Tendler

There was no question about choosing to have a natural birth for our second child. The first one had been all natural, but pretty tough and a lot of work. I figured if I could make it through all that, this one should either be the same or easier, right? I knew what to expect this time, so I felt even more confident that I would be fine. Since it was less than two years since the birth of our son, we chose not to do a birthing class this time and just listened to our relaxation meditations and music.

I started going to a chiropractor about half way through the pregnancy. My sciatica was acting up, and it was making it difficult to care for my son, Jacob. It was the best decision ever! He specialized in working with pregnancy and children, so I didn't even have to worry about childcare to go to my appointments, as my son was welcomed there as well. I would leave feeling like a million bucks and always looked forward to those days. He was also able to release tension in my ligaments and help me avoid pain there, too.

Fast forward to the third trimester—I am feeling great and really looking forward to this birth. My husband tells me that he has to go away on business for my 36th week. Great. I can't deliver at the birthing center until I get to 37 weeks anyway, so I just focus on that. He comes back and all is fine. Then he tells me he has to go to Texas for one day, right when I will be 39 weeks. UGH. I try to focus on every other day on the calendar to have this baby, but that one. The night he leaves, I have a super small tinge of blood when I went to the bathroom and think "great," but try not to think about it and go to bed. At 3:30 a.m. I wake up as usual, but my hips feel really tight, so I roll over and try to go back to sleep. It doesn't work. I get up and try to take a shower to loosen everything up. I would like to add that the tightening in my hips is happening every 6-10 minutes. I call my husband. His cell phone is off. I call his work cell, off. Now I am getting panicky. I call the hotel several times before they finally pick up the phone and get them to page his room. Finally I get to talk to him and tell him I am having contractions. UGH, this is not what we wanted. I switch back on my denial and get dressed to go to work. I feed cheerios to Jacob while I drive. I know I am still having contractions, but I am focusing on the road and driving, so I don't really feel them except for that little bit of tightness in my hips. I choose to drive by the daycare and not drop him off for the day. Jacob had been to every midwife appointment, and we had prepared him to be at the birth. Even though I was in denial about being in labor, I still kept him with me. I get to work about an hour before I normally do, still having contractions six minutes apart. We get to my office and now he needs a diaper change. Back down to the car because I forgot the diaper bag, and then back up to my office. Then I start coming back to reality. I call my boss, who also happens to be my mother-in-law and ask her to come in. I had tried to feel my cervix, but couldn't feel anything there. I figure I should get to the birthing center to find out what is really going on with this labor. It feels completely different than with my first. The birthing center is only a tenth of a mile away, so I drive over. Midwife Cathy Parisi checks me and tells me I am 7cm dilated. Crash … it all hit at once that I am having a baby right now and without my husband. I start crying and call him to let him know. There was not going to be any time for relaxation music or meditation or anything. I was having the baby now. I called my mother-in-law to bring over Jacob and make my way up to the birthing suite. Our car had been packed with all my birthing stuff since week 36, just in case. Cathy went out to wait for them and get my bag. Jacob pointed out my red bag with everything I needed, and then I get into the birthing tub. It is 8:00 a.m. The tub feels awesome and I can feel the tension in my hips relax as I squat. At 8:15 a.m. my water breaks and I can feel my body starting to push. Being in the water enabled me to move and float in whatever position I needed at that moment; it was great. Pushing was a bit more intense than last time because my nerves weren't all deadened. I could feel the baby's whole head inside my body; it was pretty cool, but sort of intimidating at the same time since I knew it was going to come out. I pushed for less than 30 minutes this time. As soon as the head came out, I had to breathe through a few contractions and not push to prevent the tearing that happened last time. That is the hardest part of the whole delivery! Finally, out came baby and right onto me. I was not tired at all and was able to fully absorb every second. They gave me my cell phone to call my husband. While on the phone with him, I checked to see if it was a boy or a girl. We had another boy!

Elijah Jayden was here. He came out in the "right" position, which is why labor was so much easier this time around, even though he weighed over a pound more than his brother. I cut the cord, and then we started working on getting out of the tub.

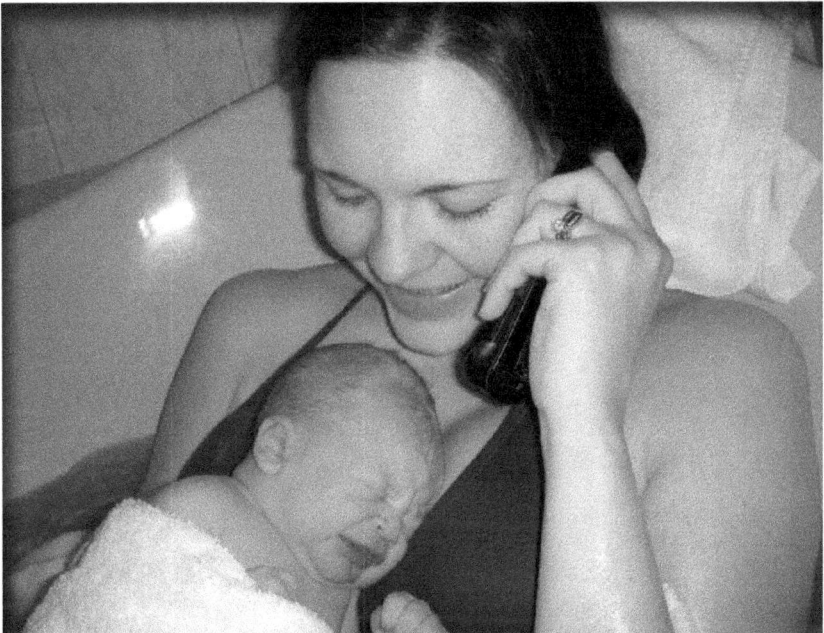

Krista sharing the joyful news with her husband after the birth of Elijah

Once we got out of the tub and into bed, we immediately started breastfeeding to get the placenta to come out. I had a little tear that Cathy was able to fix, and it didn't hurt a bit. Cathy was so good to me during the labor and delivery. She had this motherly attitude that was warm and supportive. We all knew doing this without my husband was not ideal, and she really stepped up for me by making me feel comfortable and supported. Afterwards, Jacob came in to meet his new brother. I had wanted him to actually be present for the birth, but he was more interested in playing at the time. It was cute to see his confusion about the baby no longer being in my belly anymore. Six hours later I went home. My husband came home early the next morning and finally met Elijah. I feel lucky that this labor and delivery was so much easier than the first since I didn't have my husband there for support. We are now a family of four. We are all very bonded to our newest addition and Jacob has become an amazing big brother.

6

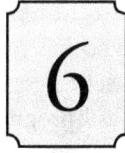

Birthing with Grace

By Sara and Grace Guenther

As I look back on our birth story, I am reminded it was the manifestation of a journey beginning with pregnancy and ending with the final contraction. Our birth story encompasses this journey.

I view pregnancy as a normal, natural, healthy process and wanted to celebrate the miracle of life growing within versus seeking out pathology. The midwifery model of care resonated with me, and I was seeking to find a midwife with whom I connected. Initially, I was leaning towards a home birth and my husband Eric was leaning towards a hospital birth. But after meeting with Tracy for a perspective client orientation at Mountain Midwifery Center in Englewood, Colorado, we were both convinced this was the place for us. Tracy, being a strong, confident, and knowledgeable woman, effectively communicated her beliefs about natural childbirth. Her enthusiasm was contagious, and we left the orientation feeling excited about pregnancy and labor/delivery. It felt so right to surround ourselves with people who believed in the process of birth and believed in me. The midwives at Mountain Midwifery Center sought to educate and empower us, rather than instill a sense of fear and anxiety.

Early in my first trimester, I started attending prenatal yoga regularly. This class would soon become so much more than merely an asana practice. With the guidance of our fearless teacher Laura, this class became a weekly support group. I was able to share my fears, anxieties, excitement, and experiences in a safe, supportive environment. Every week I had an opportunity to connect with like-minded women, who also believed in the power of birth.

During my second trimester, I started attending the Thornton/Northglenn La Leche League meetings. The first meeting I attended turned out to be transformational. I met Amy who would soon become a good friend, as well as our doula, and Karrin who has earned a very special place in our child's heart. The women at La Leche League invited me into their lives and provided much needed support as I progressed through my pregnancy, not to mention all the valuable information I received about breastfeeding and a space to be in the presence of women who were passionate about nursing their babies/toddlers/children.

Our baby, who was nicknamed Peanut, was due on January 7, 2009. As an eager first time mom, I thought Peanut would arrive either before his/her due date or shortly after. I was mistaken. Peanut was seven days late, and every day that passed I became more and more worried. Although our midwives kept assuring us that most first time moms will go 7-10 days past their due date, I still continued to worry. I was worried I would risk out and not have a chance to labor at Mountain Midwifery Center. We met with our midwife Cassie several times towards the end of my pregnancy. During the 40 week visit, Cassie said, "Sara, be prepared you may still be pregnant for another week or two. I know you want to have your baby now, but, unfortunately, you do not have control over that. You do, however, have the choice to enjoy these last couple weeks of pregnancy or live in a state of anxiety. The choice is yours." After that appointment I decided I would set my intention to savor the final couple weeks of pregnancy and be open to whatever the universe had in store for us. Much easier said than done!

At our 41–week appointment, my cervix was ripe (2.5 centimeters dilated, 70% effaced, and anteriorly positioned) and Peanut was at a -1 station. Nancy, another one of our midwives, recommended stripping my membranes. She stated if this was going to work, I would probably go into labor within 24–48 hours. Our appointment was at 2:00 p.m., and by 9:30 p.m., I was relatively sure labor was quickly approaching. I tried lying down to get some rest, but the contractions kept intensifying. At 11:30 p.m. as I was lying on the overstuffed chair in our living room, my water broke. The fluid was gushing out as I quickly made my way to the bathroom.

Nancy, our midwife on call, asked that I try to labor at home for a couple more hours. My contractions were approximately three to four minutes apart, but Nancy thought I would be more comfortable laboring at home than coming to the birth center immediately. Peanut had moved into the left occiput posterior position and I was experiencing intense back labor. I found some relief in the shower; however, the hot water only lasted for about 30 minutes, and I had to find another technique to cope with the contractions. I decided to walk around the house during contractions and utilize vocalization in an attempt to dissipate the pain. Eric, who had been diligently timing contractions, would stop and provide much needed counter pressure on my lower back.

At 2:00 a.m. Eric and I made our way to Mountain Midwifery Center. I was dreading the 30 minute car ride as I knew I would be in a confined space and unable to move around. It was during this ride, though, that I found and embraced my breath. The vocalization was not working anymore and seemed to make the contractions more intense. I would inhale through my nose and exhale audibly through my mouth as I focused on relaxing my jaw. I also closed my eyes and found one point of focus through the contraction.

At 2:30 a.m. we met our doula Amy, midwife Nancy, and midwife in training Collette at Mountain Midwifery Center. Nancy asked what room I wanted to labor in and at that point I didn't care. I just wanted to get into the tub, hoping it would alleviate my back labor. I was worried Nancy would tell me I needed to go home because I was not dilated enough, but during our first vaginal exam, I went from 3 cm to 5 cm in a matter of seconds. I then got into the tub, but to my disappointment, the back labor continued.

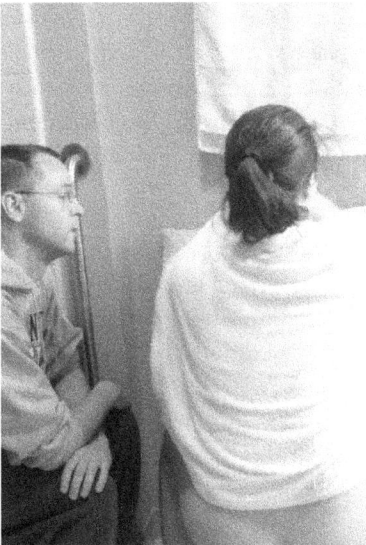

Eric supporting Sara as she labored

For the next four hours, I would alternate from the tub, to sitting backwards on the toilet, to walking around the birth center, to utilizing distraction techniques. I even tried horse lips, spiraling my body to connect with the energy of the contractions, and, of course, continued to focus on my breath. No matter what technique I utilized the back labor did not pass, not even between contractions, but eventually I surrendered to the sensations. Through the support of my compassionate husband, our midwives, and doula, I was able to be present in the moment, but also be an observer to the process.

Throughout my labor I would find myself shaking, sometimes uncontrollably. Initially, I was confused as to why I kept shaking, but now believe it was my body's way of coping with the intensity of labor.

Around 6:00–6:30 a.m., Nancy and Collette left and Tracy arrived. Tracy started to work her magic immediately. She presented options in a way that gave me a choice, yet motivated me to move and try new positions. I tried squatting at the squatting stool for a few contractions, and also spiraled my body as I let a sling hung from the ceiling support me.

Eventually, I found my way back into the tub and was pushing. Tracy kept saying, "We deliver babies from our butt, not from our vagina." This was her comical way of encouraging me to push in a way that was familiar to me. I found myself pushing with such strength and determination that I screamed and wailed during most pushes to release pent up energy and to open up. Around 7:50 a.m., Tracy said, "I bet you will have your baby by 8:00 a.m." I immediately doubted her and thought she was trying to give me false hope.

At approximately 7:56 a.m., Tracy said, "You can stay in the tub if you like, but if you get out of the tub, you will have your baby quicker." That was all I needed to hear. I immediately started to get out of the tub while Gina, our nurse, started to place chux pads around the squatting stool and Tracy was starting to put her gloves on. Suddenly Gina yelled, "Tracy, you need to catch this baby NOW!" The act of getting out of the tub was all that was needed for our baby to literally slide right out.

I started crying uncontrollably as Tracy placed our baby in my arms. I didn't even think to look to see if we were blessed with a daughter or a son. I just couldn't believe our baby had arrived and my back labor was gone. Eric finally said, "It's a girl!" Grace was born at 7:58 a.m., two minutes before 8:00 a.m., just as Tracy had predicted.

Laura, my prenatal yoga teacher once said, "We labor like we live our lives." This couldn't have been truer for me. I doubted myself and was unsure if I could do it, but throughout the entire process I labored on. I was determined and committed to doing it naturally and never questioned that decision. I would be lying if I said labor wasn't painful. It was extremely painful as Grace moved from left occiput posterior to right occiput posterior, and eventually moved into a right anterior position. Labor was the most physically, emotionally, and spiritually challenging thing I have ever done, but also the most transformational and life enhancing. I am blessed for having had this experience, and now have a precious daughter who is a manifestation of this journey.

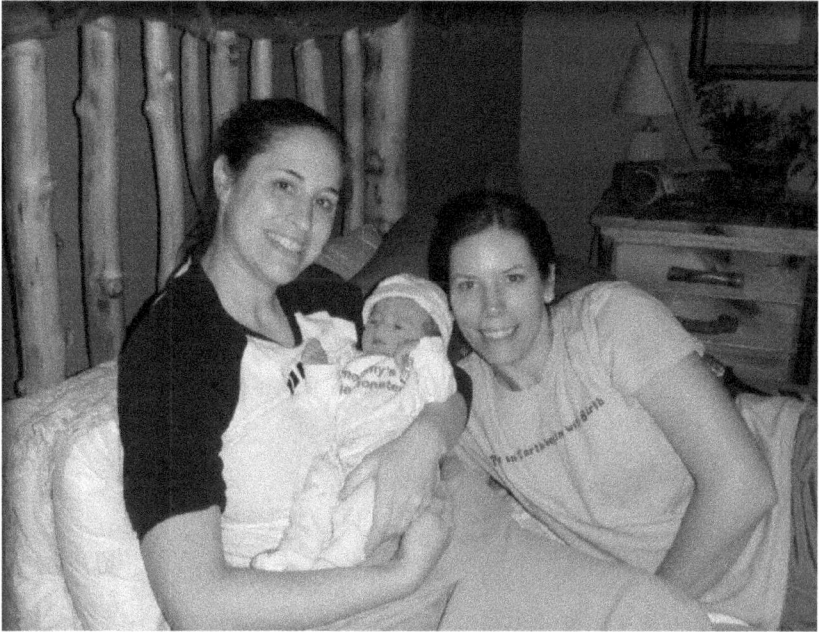

Sara holding baby Grace after the birth with midwife Tracy

I am grateful to my husband, our midwives, our doula, my prenatal yoga teacher, all the pregnant women whom I met throughout the journey, and to our family and friends for their encouragement, support, and friendship. Most of all, I am grateful to Grace for embarking on this journey with me and for being my greatest teacher. Together, Grace and I created a birth story that demonstrates the health and beauty of pregnancy, labor, and delivery, but also the reality of the challenges and inner journey of childbirth. Together, we were able to birth with Grace!

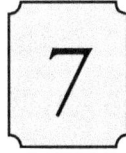

7

Natural and Nurtured

By Miranda Pacchiana

When I gave birth to my son Jackson in a birthing center, I was already a mother. My first child was born 18 months earlier in a traditional hospital. Elated and grateful as I was to have delivered a healthy, beautiful daughter, I realized as time passed that the hospital model was not the right fit for our family. For our second birth, my husband and I wanted things to be different.

During our first child's birth, the hospital had given me Pitocin to speed up my labor (seemingly for no reason other than their convenience), precipitating the need for an epidural to stem the pain of my extremely strong contractions. Once Emma was born, she was immediately bathed, given eye drops and an injection in her foot, all while she screamed in obvious discomfort. Only when she was finally swaddled and placed in my arms did she quiet down, at which point my husband and I could relax and truly celebrate our new child. The experience left me wishing the hospital staff had a better understanding of my baby's needs, as well as policies that showed respect for a woman's natural birthing abilities.

Jackson's birth turned out to be everything we had been looking for. While pregnant with him, I learned that a birthing center had just opened nearby. I knew as soon as I met the two midwives and toured the brand-new birthing rooms that they had created a place which strived to give families the type of birth I had been envisioning. The comfortable atmosphere gave me the feeling of being a welcome guest in a beautiful, newly built home. There was a tasteful kitchen open to a family room, and two nicely decorated bedrooms. Both birthing rooms had rocking chairs, real beds, and large master bathrooms, with showers and oversized bathtubs. Hidden in an armoire was emergency equipment, and the hospital was just across the street in case anything went wrong. This was important to us because as much as we wanted a relaxed, natural experience, we needed reassurance that our baby would have access to high-tech medical care if necessary.

On the day I went into labor, my husband Adam and I arrived at the birthing center at 8:00 a.m. I was only two centimeters dilated, so the midwife on call sent me home until things progressed. Back home, I spent time with my daughter and my mother, who had come over to baby sit for the day. In my relaxed state, the contractions really began to pick up. After only an hour, we were back in the car again and on our way to deliver our second child. I remember how uncomfortable every bump in the road felt, but Adam carefully pulled over each time I indicated a particularly strong contraction.

Cathy, the midwife who would deliver Jackson, had just come on call, and she examined me once we arrived. This time I was dilated five centimeters. For the next couple of hours, Cathy and Adam and I waited out my labor together. We chatted between contractions and I was allowed to drink and eat lightly. I got in the bathtub and munched on a bagel. Pretty soon, I was seven centimeters dilated. The contractions were getting quite painful, but Cathy coached me through them. In my state of discomfort, she knew intuitively how to encourage me without agitating me further. She described what my body was doing and reminded me that the pain was moving me toward the ultimate goal of meeting my baby. Adam rubbed my lower back where the pain seemed to be concentrated. Increasingly uncomfortable, I decided to take a shower, and I squatted down as the warm water ran over me. Eventually, Cathy told me that I had been at seven centimeters for quite some time, and she suggested that I allow her to break my bag of waters. Feeling tired and eager to speed up the process, I agreed.

As soon as she broke my water, waves of very intense contractions swept over me. I was really in pain, but it was different than the labor I had experienced with Pitocin. These contractions were not unmanageable. With the emotional support of my calm, encouraging midwife and husband, I knew I could handle it. As I squatted on the floor and shifted my weight from side to side, Cathy encouraged me to make a low, moaning sound. Leaving behind my inhibitions, I did as she said as I listened to her words of approval, breaking through the pain that seemed to envelop me.

Suddenly, I realized that I wanted to get on all fours and I climbed onto the bed. Cathy asked me if I wanted to give birth there. "I don't know," I told her, feeling unable to process a logical decision in my painful state. And then I wanted to push. The nurse prepared the bed with a sterile covering while Adam stayed close, excitedly encouraging me on. After only seven minutes of pushing, the baby's head emerged. Cathy had intentionally positioned Adam in the center of the action and now he watched as our baby, the rest of his body still inside me, opened his eyes and looked around. Cathy asked Adam what it looked like, and he told us, "I think it's a boy!"

With one more push, Jackson came out, right into Adam's hands. It was a perfect moment when I heard my husband tell me himself that we had a baby boy. I heard his little cry, and I rolled over and held Jackson in my arms. He was beautiful and alert. I loved him completely.

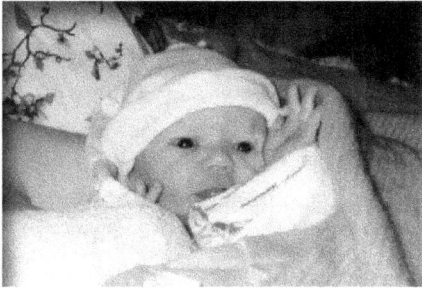

Baby Jackson just born

The next few hours were spent exactly as I had hoped. I lay in bed with Adam as we admired our precious new son. The setting was peaceful; the mood was celebratory. Cathy's sincerity was obvious as she told us that we were a great team during labor, and we felt proud of ourselves. I was encouraged to breastfeed as soon as I was ready, and the post-partum nurse cheerfully told me that I appeared to have excellent equipment for the job. This was a marked contrast to the negative message I'd gotten from the hospital nurses after my first birth, who told me that my fair skin meant I would probably have sore breasts. Jackson nursed beautifully. With his natural, waxy coating, he felt soft and smelled absolutely delicious. I remember thinking this was nature's way of making him even more appealing to his parents. I asked the nurse if she intended to bathe him, and she said no, that, in fact, this coating was protective, and she discouraged me from washing him for at least a day or two.

It was early evening when, about four hours later, we dressed Jackson in a bunting and packed up to go home. Sitting next to my baby in the car, it felt funny to see his tiny body scrunched into a car seat, knowing that just hours before he had been safely inside my womb. The half-hour trip felt very long, as I yearned to take my baby back in my arms and to see my daughter.

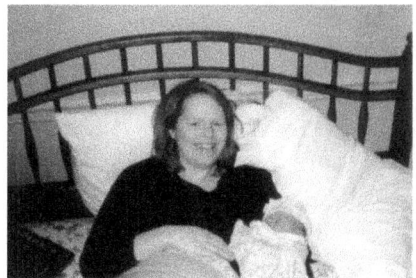

Miranda with baby Jackson

It was a joyous homecoming. My mother greeted us excitedly and stole a peek at her new grandson as Adam quietly brought him upstairs. My daughter Emma and I had never been separated for an entire day before, and we had a happy reunion, as she proudly told me what she and Nana had done together that day. Finally, I casually asked her if she would like to meet her new baby brother. She jumped up excitedly, and I led her and my mother upstairs. Right away, Emma asked to hold him. We told her how proud we were of her, that she was a big sister now, and she beamed as she examined her brother's tiny face. My mother watched the scene before her with great delight and admiration for the serene manner in which we had allowed it to unfold.

We consider ourselves truly fortunate that Jackson's labor and delivery experience was an ideal one for our family. We felt the sacredness of our baby's birth was honored by the staff of the birthing center. Jackson greatly benefited because nature was allowed to take its course in every aspect of the process. In the quiet setting, he met his parents and made his entrance into the outside world in peace. He was swaddled and cuddled, surrounded by an atmosphere of good will and respect for our family's needs. I felt pleased to discover that my body could go into labor and push my baby out on its own. After the birth, I was tired and sore, but much less so than the first time around when I'd had to contend with medicine forcing my body into labor too intensely. In pictures right after Jackson was born, I actually look pretty good, and the elation on my face is obvious. Emma benefited, too, by meeting her brother in her own home and seeing her happy parents so soon after the delivery. For all of these reasons, Adam and I highly recommend a birthing center experience for other parents and their babies.

8

A Dream Comes True: My Birth Story

By Kristin Afdahl

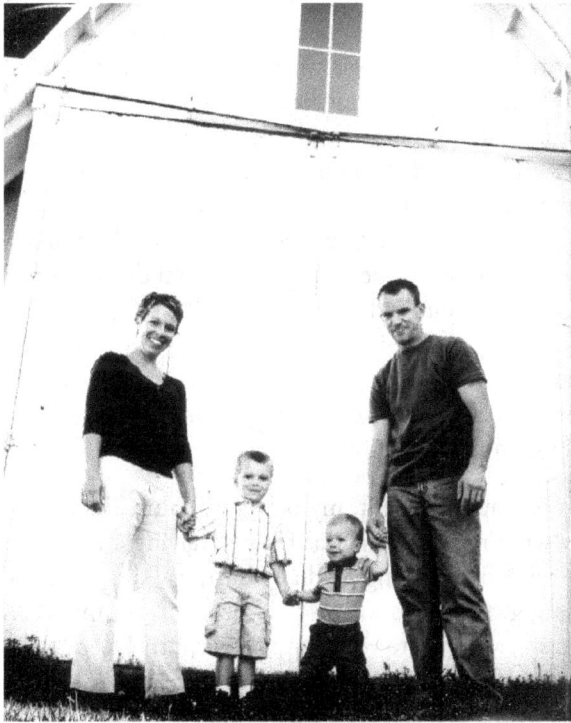

The Afdahl family: Kristen, Bo, Ian and Brad

Most girls dream about their wedding day. Don't get me wrong, I certainly did enough of that! But what I also dreamt about was having a baby. Birth always fascinated me. You see, I grew up on a farm watching many animals give birth. I'd sit there and watch from beginning to end. I'd really study the mother and how she walked around and around during contractions. And how she'd push and bellow, and how "traumatic" it seemed to me at the time. Then it was like a light switch flipped when the calf was born. She was quiet and still, and in awe with her new calf. It was always so amazing to me how females of any kind can carry offspring. It's just such a miracle, how the body is designed to do that. Then I found *Our bodies, Ourselves: A Book By and For Women* by The Boston Women's Health Book Collective in my mom's book collection, and I was even more amazed. In it there was a photo of a woman giving birth. That was it, I was hooked. I wanted to have a baby someday—just like that. Naturally. And I wanted to have my husband there with me, and to feel that love for my newborn, just like those mother cows did for their calves.

I have two children. My first birth experience was good, normal by most standards, just not something I'd want to do again. I had a great pregnancy, loving every bit of it, and I really felt good. My son Bo was born in a hospital. I thought since it was my first birth, I'd better play it safe and give birth where "society" thought I should. I labored for eight hours, mostly in a tub of warm water, which was wonderful. I did have a birth plan—no drugs were on that plan. I told my husband, no matter how bad it got, I did not want drugs. At one point I did ask for drugs. Yes, I caved in, but he stood strong and reminded me of my wish. When I felt like pushing, I remember the nurses saying, "No, wait, let me check you first." OK, so she did and said, "You are at a 10, let's get you out of the tub now." WHAT? Out of the tub? You see at the time, my hospital didn't birth babies in the water, so I had to get out and birth on the table. Well, try walking or even standing after hours of pushing, being physically exhausted, and then don't forget the baby down in your pelvis. Not easy. After getting onto the table, I pushed, and with the help of a vacuum, my baby was out. It was too much, too fast, and very painful.

At my two-week appointment, my pelvis still hurt. Being my first child, I didn't know what normal pain was for just having a baby two weeks ago. But this hurt was bad. Lifting my baby hurt, walking hurt, going up steps was excruciating, getting into the car hurt, putting my socks on was an impossible task, even just to touch my pelvis hurt. Deep in my heart, I felt there was something wrong, but after hearing, "It's just all in your head" from the doctor, I put it aside. Maybe it was all in my head?

But the pain continued, and after thinking about it, I realized that I had this same pain the last few months of my pregnancy, too. I thought it was normal to feel that pressure and pelvic pain. So, I started doing some research on my own. What I discovered I had was pretty common and was called Symphysis Pubic Dysfunction. Pretty big word for what essentially means pelvic pain. Birthsource.com gave this description, "This pain is a result of separation of the symphysis pubis, which is a joint in the very front part of the pelvic bone structure. There is cartilage that fills the gap in the bones. During pregnancy, hormones, such as relaxin, soften this cartilage, allowing the pelvic bones to be more flexible for delivery. Some women, however, have too much play in the pelvis, causing a large gap between the bones. This makes the symphysis pubis area extremely sensitive to touch." I found a lot of articles online about SPD.

After about two years, I still had pain, but not as severe. I knew now how to walk up steps without pain and how to get into and out of the car. The scary part was that I wanted to have another child. My main concern was what if the pain was intensified or what if I damaged the area even worse? I knew I had to go a more natural, health-based route. I needed someone to listen to me and not tell me it "was all in my head." That's when I spoke with a midwife, Paula Bernini Feigal, CPM, in Menomonie, Wisconsin, at Morning Star Birth Center. I had called her and asked if she had ever heard of this problem, and she said that she had heard of it, but hadn't had too many people with the condition. Still, she was happy to work with me to have a safe and natural birth just as I wanted. Well, that was what I wanted to hear. I had found someone who would listen and care for me.

Within two months of finding Paula, I was pregnant. Guess it was meant to be! This was great. I was excited to feel good again. This time I wanted to do it differently, and after meeting with Paula, I knew a midwife was the plan for me. I never had fear of birthing naturally. I've always known that a woman's body is designed to give birth, and that fear would only get in the way of birth. I had actually wanted to birth at my home, but my husband thought it'd be best to go to the birth center since it was only 30 minutes from our home and only two minutes from a hospital in case things didn't go as planned. I agreed. Sometimes I get too opinionated, and this time I had to compromise.

The birth center was terrific. There were two rooms, and we could choose which one we wanted to deliver in. Each was comfortably decorated, just like my home, and both had large tubs and private bathrooms. I also created a new birth plan, describing each and every detail of what my dream birth would be.

During my pregnancy, my SPD did come back. I was pretty uncomfortable. I focused on chiropractic care to make sure my pelvis was in place. I also had the wonderful help from my midwife. She had me wear a V-Belt. It was odd looking, kind of like a jock strap. It was designed to be real tight to keep everything in the pelvic region in place. After putting it on, I could have cared less what it or I looked like wearing it, it was heaven. I just wore it right over my underwear literally for months, even at night in the last few months.

At 38 weeks I was pretty ready to give birth. When August came, I felt like any day would be the day. I was so excited. I knew relief from the SPD would only happen entirely if the baby was out and not putting pressure on my pelvis. So, I was ready for the baby to be out!

August 17th was a gorgeous summer night. I had just fallen asleep when I felt a "snap" in my pelvis, the weirdest thing. Now I know it was my water breaking. As I walked to the bathroom, I leaked all the way there, and when I sat on the toilet, I leaked more and urinated at the same time. Even though it was my second child, I was still wondering, "Was that pee or did my water just break?" I didn't have any contractions … yet. I called my midwife to let her know what was happening. She said to call her back when the contractions started. In the meantime, we called my mother-in-law to come and watch our three-year-old while we were gone. About 30 minutes later, the contractions started and didn't stop. They were right on top of another, so we quickly prepared to head to the birth center. My contractions were two minutes apart. When my mother-in-law arrived at about 11:00 p.m., I couldn't talk or walk through the contractions, so things were pretty intense. I did cry when she walked in the door. For a brief minute, I "lost it" and let all my emotions go. I was excited and scared to death all in one moment. That moment was one I knew would be a last. I thought about my little boy who was sleeping in his bed, and I knew that when he woke up he would have a sibling. He wouldn't be the only child anymore, my only child. But I had told myself we had gone through all of this with him. He was excited to have a brother or sister, and he knew that some morning if he woke up and mama and daddy weren't there that we were off to have the baby. So, after my brief breakdown, I concentrated on this new life that was to come out and greet us (any second it felt like).

We raced to the center, but it felt like an eternity getting there, and every bump was pretty painful. The entire way I had my eyes shut, just hoping when I next opened them we'd be there. I felt it easier to focus on what was happening inside my body if I had my eyes shut, plus Brad was going so fast that I thought I'd get carsick if I looked out the window! I put the seat all the way back and just had my belly hanging between my legs.

My husband was so wonderful through the entire labor and birth. He has always been my total support, my best friend. This night was no different. As I walked into the birth center, the first things I heard was, "Kristin, we have the blue room ready for you and your bath is drawn." They knew me, they knew the room I wanted, and they knew I wanted to give birth in the water. It was going perfectly as planned! Paula, the midwife, checked my cervix and I was dilated to a 4. I then got in the tub and talk about heaven! Until another contraction started, anyway. But between the contractions, I was able to relax with the warm water and stare at the changing colored lights on the side of the tub. They were perfectly sequenced in time, changing about every minute or so into a different color. It was so relaxing. I was more drawn to the blue and green lights, so I was always looking forward to them coming back on. It was a great calming distraction from the contractions. My husband was the biggest help, just being there through it all, sitting at the edge of the tub or helping me in and out if I needed to go to the bathroom. He was there for me to talk to or cry to, or squeeze when the contractions came. I think in the end, my job was easier than his!

Things went very fast once I was in the tub, and I soon felt the overwhelming urge to push. I asked Paula if this could be happening so soon, I had only been there at the center for 30 minutes. She said to listen to my body and if I needed to push to push. This was a much different message than I remembered from my first birth—"don't push until we get you on the table." It was great feeling, like I was in control this time.

I'll admit it—every contraction was pretty intense. I didn't get a break between them. It was pretty constant, but I calmed myself down knowing that this is the only way to get the baby out. I knew my body was pushing its hardest to do this for me; I had to stay in a relaxed and focused state of mind to let it do its job. It's almost as if I was in a trance. Moaning and swearing and being as loud as I wanted felt good. I remember a few breaks between the contractions. It was so quiet.

Paula had a great team. She had two women training to be midwifes that night. Krista was there, with encouraging words, and Erin, with her homemade paper fan, fanning me off when I said I was dizzy and hot. Everyone was there, right by my side, but very quiet, listening to my needs. I remember the windows of the bathroom being open, and it being so darn hot (the AC wasn't working that day), but that quiet brought a sense of calm over me to know that with the next contraction I could do it. That is what I just kept telling myself, "I can do it," over and over and over and over. So, I was ready, I was ready to push, and given the "go ahead," I started. I remember Paula saying to reach down and feel my baby's head. I felt the bag of water, and at that instant, it broke in my hand. I then felt my baby's head, and with one more push, he was out. I reached down and brought him out of the water onto my chest. He was just beautiful. What a perfect experience.

72   Spontaneous Joyful Natural Birth

He didn't breath right away, which was a bit scary for me, but Paula was in control the entire time. She just flicked his feet a few times, and he started breathing normally. She covered him with a warm blanket and laid him on my chest. After my placenta was done pulsing, Brad cut the cord and he was free. The funniest part of the whole thing was this: I didn't even look to see what sex the baby was. I was so tired and glad it was all over and that I had this beautiful baby, that it took me a bit to look down and realize it was a boy!

Ian David Afdahl was born at 12:58 a.m., August 18th, 2007. It was a significantly different birth than my first, only three hours of labor and two pushes and I had a beautiful baby. The biggest difference was that I got to do it how I wanted and that is how it is supposed to be—natural, without any interventions, feeling in control.

At three weeks postpartum, I felt great. Knowing that SPD can cause pain for weeks or even years after a birth, I opted to take charge of my pelvic health this time and worked with a chiropractor who specialized in women's health. She made sure that my pelvis was moving back to where it should be after Ian's birth and healing properly. I felt so great taking charge of my pelvic health this time around, choosing to give birth in the water, squatting, letting my baby come out naturally, and choosing to work with a chiropractor and midwife immediately after my delivery. All of those things helped with me with the SPD, but can also be so wonderful for any healthy woman who wants a successful birth experience. I also believe taking Omega 3 Fish Oil supplements throughout my pregnancy helped tremendously with postpartum blues. After my first consultation with my midwife, she recommended this supplement after I had told her about my terrible two-week postpartum blues with my first child. Since I already knew Omega 3 would be good for the baby's brain development, I felt I had nothing to lose. Maybe it could help me, too? And it did.

My goal is to help make women knowledgeable about SPD. Women need to know that pelvic pain is not normal during and after birth, and there are things you can do to help yourself. Now, three years after my last pregnancy, my pelvis is in better shape than ever. Knowledge is key—key to anything in life. Fear is lack of knowledge. I believe that if you know why your body is doing what it is doing, then you should have no fear, just let it get its job done and let your mind be in control. Even with all of the support you may have, it's YOU that has to birth the baby, YOU that has to be strong and overcome lots of emotions, fears, and most of all—yes, I'll say it, pain. Birthing naturally is an empowering experience. It's something you'll take with you forever and never forget.

9

Brendan's and Gabrielle's Birth

By Monique Drury

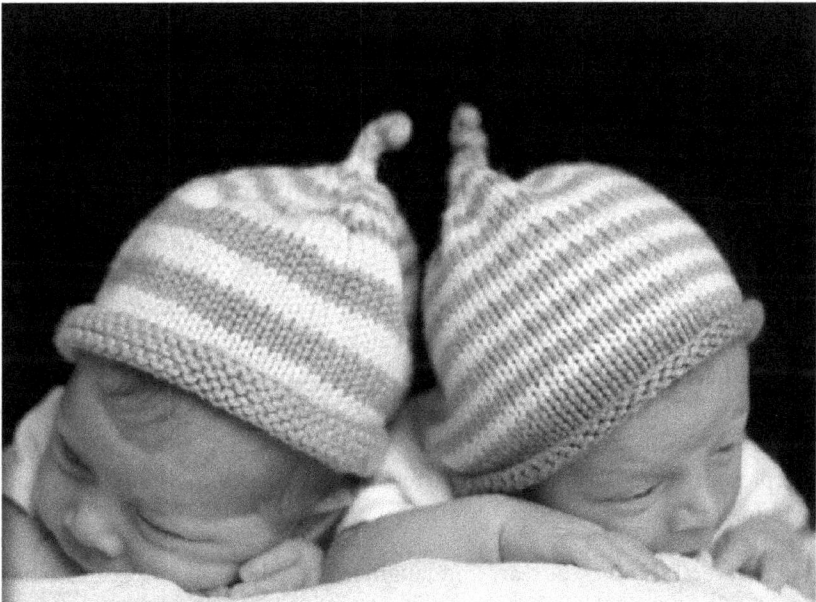

Brendan and Gabrielle

At 20 weeks, we went for our first ultrasound. As I waited for Brad to arrive, the ultrasound technician suggested that we get some routine measurements out of the way. She would be sure to wait for his arrival to determine the gender of the baby. So, we got started.

As images of head, spine, and femur flashed across the screen, the tech began to shift uncomfortably in her chair. She seemed hesitant and kept flicking her glance toward me, as if she wanted to say something. Worry washed over me. Is there something wrong? Then she suddenly blurted out, "I just have to tell you ... there are *two* babies in here." My jaw dropped. Brad walked in. He stopped dead in his tracks at the sight of my face. Through tears and laughter, I broke the news to Brad—we were having twins!

He smiled. I vacillated between sheer panic and overwhelming excitement. We were already halfway through the pregnancy (and behind on every project), and suddenly we were expecting two babies!

Now we had some news to share. We called our daughter Amber. Slyly, we gave her one last shot to guess—boy or girl. "Girl," she guessed. We told her that she was half right. She stuttered and stammered ... and then she got it. A boy and a girl.

Our next stop was the Green House Birth Center (GBC) for our 20–week appointment. Brad had a bone to pick with Clarice. Rewind to week 16, Brad had been tempting the wrath of pregnant women everywhere by telling me that I was "getting pretty big." I figured that it was just because it was my second pregnancy. Week 12 was normal. At week 16, I measured a little big according to our midwife Clarice. I joked, "not twins big, right?" She said, "Oh, no, no." Brad looked skeptical. I shrugged it off; I measured big with Alex, too.

As soon as we walked into the GBC, Brad 'confronted' Clarice. I am sure that she puts him solidly into the category of rascal. Their interaction generally entails poking of fun and sage playful admonishing. There was a new family settling in after a recent birth. Everyone was there. Brad in his most convincing tone scolded Clarice for not warning us. She looked perplexed. Twins. Clarice uncharacteristically yelled out, "Holy s***!" and wrapped me into a big hug.

After several minutes of tears and laughter, the talk went straight to what-am-I-gonna-do?!? The GBC had intentionally not taken twin or breech births in the past, so as not to stir the political pot. Our midwives, Kip and Clarice, looked at each other, and then at Brad and me. We all knew that I had to birth there—safe, comfortable, and familiar. Since the GBC had established a solid reputation, the midwives had been considering the idea of twin birth, and this might be the right time. Of course, it was. I have learned that everything happens the way that it should. I had no reservations. I knew that I was strong, healthy, and prepared to give birth at the GBC.

Truthfully, I was terrified of being at the hospital with all of those drugs and scalpels, and hands just itching to use them.

So, it was settled. Barring any complications, I was to deliver my babies in the most ideal setting with the best attendants I could imagine. As a back-up measure, I was to set-up concurrent care with Dr. Nancy Herta, a wonderful obstetrician and a GBC mom herself.

The next few months went by without a hitch. And then I got big and fast! Not just big—we are talking can't-find-a-circus-tent-big-enough-to-cover-my-belly big. I measured 47.5 inches *around*—that is nearly 4 feet! I am 5'2" tall. I was tired. I was ornery. I was uncomfortable … all the time.

Thirty-five weeks came and went. Then 36 and 37 weeks. Whew! I had made it. Our little girl finally decided to stay head-down, along with her brother who had been vertex since our ultrasound. They were developing beautifully. He was my rowdy boy and determined to come first. She was my tranquil girl; I would patiently wait for a gentle wiggle or nudge from her.

Then halfway through my 37th week, as I fought my nightly duel with insomnia, something happened … my water broke. It was Sunday morning about 1:15 a.m. Brad woke as if he knew something subconsciously. I told him that I thought my water had broken. It still didn't seem real.

I proceeded to pack a bag and we hurriedly discussed names. I reminded him that Kip would not let us leave without names for the babies. We felt really unprepared. We called the midwives to let them know my water had broken.

About an hour later, the first contraction came … without training wheels. There were no gentle warm-up contractions. No going back to sleep for a few hours. It was business—right now. They started out eight minutes apart and came hard. They quickly dropped to six minutes apart.

I got into the shower. The hot water was sweet relief. My brain left my body. The contractions kept coming, fast and hard, with no break in between, just a lower intensity of continuous spasm. Time had no meaning. I had been in the shower for 20 minutes. My contractions were two to three minutes apart. Brad had called the midwives again; he knew I was progressing very quickly. He called to me in the shower that maybe we should get going. Although I could hear something in his voice that sounded a bit like urgency, it did not compute. I thought that I would stay in the warm soothing water for just one more …

I summoned the will to leave that blessed shower and haphazardly got dressed. My contractions were rocking me; it was all I could do to just breathe through them.

I staggered out to the van. Amber poked her head out to say goodbye. I am quite sure that I looked like a crazed animal, alternating between pacing wildly around the van and leaning on it panting. I felt like I was on a runaway train. This labor took me by surprise after the long, slow, gradual labor with Alex. I suddenly realized that I had better get on board, so I could keep up with this break-neck pace, and not just get dragged down the tracks.

Brad came out. It was time to go. It was a cool night. I started to put on my sweater and got hit by a Saharan heat wave. Oh boy, here we go! I climbed into the van. The sweater hanging off one arm, all disheveled. I knew immediately that I did not want to be in that van! Brad and I looked at each other. It was the opening day of deer season. I said to Brad, "Please take it easy. Don't hit any deer." He was thinking we should have left 30 minutes ago.

I spent the next 25 minutes letting Brad know that I wanted, *needed,* had to get out of that van! I considered climbing into the back, so I could at least get on my hands and knees. Not happening. Almost there.

We, of course, made it to the GBC because Brad was great under pressure. I walked in and Clarice met me in the hallway. I collapsed into a huge hug, as another contraction shook me. The intensity was amazing me, but it still did not occur to me that things were happening so fast.

We went into the Peach room. Our room. I looked at the giant inviting tub with trepidation. I promised myself that I would not get in until I was really ready to give birth. After 38 hours of labor with Alex, I didn't want to jump the gun. It had been less than two hours since my first contraction. It was not occurring to me that this labor was on a different cadence.

It was 4:00 a.m., less than two hours from the onset of my labor. Everything was whirling around me, with moments of vivid clarity that gave in to the blur of worldly momentum.

I remember …

Pacing in the Peach room.

Deciding that it felt right to get into the water.

That luscious hot water.

Brad being close by my side.

Kip quietly knitting.

Thinking, why is everyone in the room already? They must know something.

Focusing on letting go.

Everything fell into place. I was intentionally and fully there. I caught up with that runaway train. I was onboard and in touch with every sensation. Ready. The rhythm felt familiar and perfect.

I wavered for a moment. My mantra, 'This is hard' slipped out as 'This hurts.' I quickly corrected my thoughts and my words. I remember Kip reassuring me that *this is hard*. And yet so easy.

I closed my eyes. My mind opened—sublime. My body moved without the necessity of thought. I remember feeling my little boy descending, ready to come into the world. I narrated so everyone could know and so I could absorb the moment. He came without any effort from me. The more I relaxed, the easier it was. Just allowing the natural reflex to happen. And there he was. Perfection. Immediately, Clarice assisted him into my arms. He came into the world quickly and quietly. He was born at 5:00 a.m. on the dot.

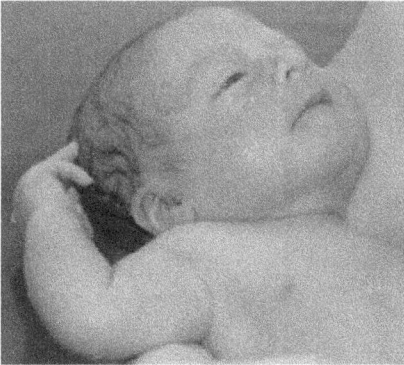

Brendan

I held him. We got to know each other. He looked around. Still not a peep. We had an appropriate amount of time to get acquainted. Then he got to meet Daddy. Daddy held him for a good amount of time. Meanwhile, I began to feel some little quakes that resembled the beginnings of a contraction.

Audra and Patrice (midwives) had shown up at some point after Brendan arrived. Now everyone was here, but one, and she was letting us know her arrival was imminent. The pace was slow and gradual. I worried aloud that it would be too slow. I wanted her to hurry up, so we could all just be together!

I didn't have to worry; she came when she was supposed to ... 6:26 a.m. My labor progressed steadily, and yes, it was a second labor. I had false hopes that the work was already done. Daddy handed Brendan to Heather, a GBC friend and birth-mom to twins herself, who rocked him close-by.

Brendan finally spoke up as my labor transitioned; he responded to my voice. Amazing.

Right before Gabrielle was born, I felt the urge to change positions from kneeling to a reclined position. I followed. She came out squawking. My tranquil little girl ... Clarice lifted her to my belly. That is as far as she could come because of a very short umbilical cord. Intuition.

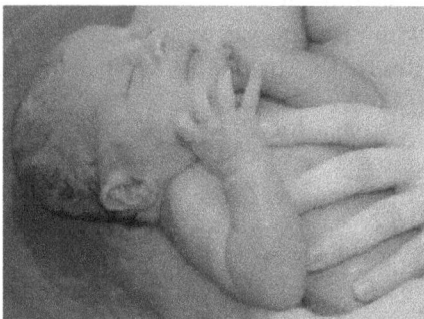

Gabrielle

Gabrielle let us know of her displeasure with the cold, new surroundings and quickly curled into my belly, and then quieted.

They were here. Two perfect little beings.

The next few hours Brad and I juggled babies and cooed and beamed. The babies nursed with ease. Brendan had been so patient, waiting for sissy to arrive. Two brand-new lives so exquisitely designed. As the four of us cuddled in bed, we noted Brendan's and Gabrielle's similarities and differences. We took them in. Every detail. Every breath.

Then Grandma and Grandpa Labadie came with Amber and Alex. It seemed like an eternity since we had seen them. It had only been a couple of hours. Alex had seemed to grow up in just that time. Alex had a cautious, curious look, and then he poured into the room and piled into bed with us. Amber was the old pro—big sis for the third time. We went about introducing everyone, and there was more baby juggling. The midwives got in on it, fussing and fawning over the babies. Pictures and more pictures. What utter joy.

It was getting toward mid-day. We wrapped up the official stuff. Brendan Robert, born at 5:00 a.m., 6 lb. 4 oz., and Gabrielle Brooke, born at 6:26 a.m., 6 lb. 12 oz. We hugged and kissed and thanked our wonderful friends for helping us welcome these two precious souls into the world. Then we headed home to rest.

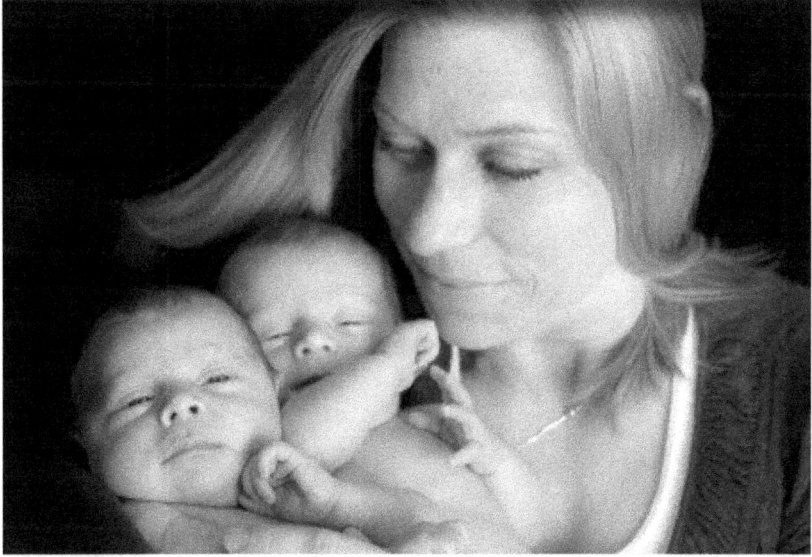

Monique, Brendan, and Gabrielle

10

The Story of Ana

By Sara Brown

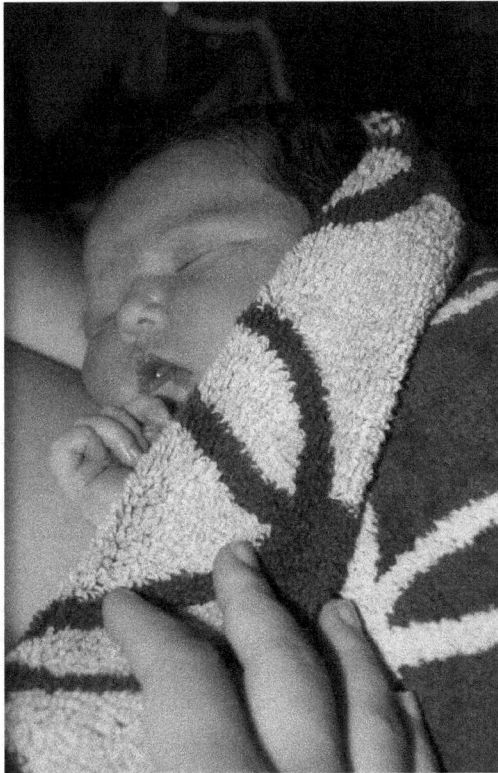

Baby Ana

Natural birth is a peaceful and very empowering experience. I felt like I could conquer the world when all was said and done. I had desired natural childbirth with my first two children, and while I did end up with two healthy, beautiful babies through vaginal deliveries, I did not have two natural births. Both were accompanied by pressure to progress faster, epidural, and pushing my babies out while lying flat on my back in a hospital bed. I felt like a patient, as I made important decisions about vaccines and pacifiers and breastfeeding. I was aware that things could be different, but I didn't know how.

When I got pregnant with our third child, I set out to discover natural birth and what that meant for me. A change in our insurance coverage forced us to look into different options. When I heard about Morning Star Birthing Center in St. Louis Park, MN, we had our answer. We had briefly discussed a home birth, with an attending midwife, but found it hard to make the jump from hospital to home. However, I also knew that if I were in a hospital, even with a midwife, I would be tempted to choose drugs. It was not ultimately what I wanted, but I knew it would stay in the back of my mind.

As the reality set in, I was scared at times. Mostly about being 40 minutes away from the birth center and delivering on the car ride there.

Would I be able to take the pain? What if something went wrong? What if my baby was too big? (My first daughter had been over nine pounds.) But the midwives were professional and ever reassuring throughout the pregnancy. They encouraged me to become educated about the birth I wanted, and provided classes and other resources.

Pretty early on in my pregnancy, I was advised to read *Ina May's Guide to Childbirth* by Ina May Gaskin. I read it again at the tail end of pregnancy and it helped so much! I took comfort in the stories the women told. I felt reassured that I was in capable hands. I remember reading one story specifically where the baby's shoulders got stuck coming out. Ina May explained how the best possible position for a mother with this issue was to be on all fours on the floor. This opened the pelvis up and allowed the baby to be born.

I also read a little on the concept of Hypnobirthing. I would imagine myself in labor and would will myself to relax every muscle and breathe deeply. The calmer I was, the quicker the baby would be born. I also learned that the body experiences more pain when tense and distressed. I decided meditation would my drug of choice this time!

It was exciting to pick the room where my baby would be born at the birth center. When I would pray and visualize the day, I would picture that room. It was also fun to get the children involved in the process and see their excitement growing. Every step of the way, care was taken to know my body. I believed prevention was key to truly knowing me and my pregnancy. We discussed diet and weight gain in a way that was so foreign to my OB/hospital experiences.

On the morning of Monday, July 19, 2010, my body began its process. All my babies had been around two weeks early, and all had started with days of contractions, starting and stopping. It was frustrating to wait and the suspense was almost more than I could bear. Finally on Friday afternoon, the 23rd, the contractions intensified, and I knew this was the time. I called my husband Dan and our midwife Paula, and arranged for childcare. I took a shower and breathed through some intense contractions. The car ride was bumpy and felt incredibly long. It was such a relief to get to the birth center and be greeted at the door by Paula. She hugged me and said excitedly, "Are you ready to have your baby today?"

We settled in and Paula checked me. I was only at 4 cm and was a little discouraged. For as much pain and intensity as I was experiencing, I was hoping to be farther along. They filled the tub and I sank in. This was such a relief! I settled into a rhythm. I concentrated hard on physically relaxing every muscle in my body, which would help me progress. I imagined my cervix opening wide to allow the baby to be born. We put music on quietly to have something to take my mind off the pain. It was late afternoon and I remember the sun shining on the water in the tub.

Our doula joined us. I had decided pretty last minute to invite her to attend our birth. She was logging hours before becoming a certified doula and was looking for births to attend. I was nervous that my husband would be out of town when I went into labor, as he travels a lot for work, and felt a doula would be a good solution for extra support. What I didn't realize was how vital she would be to the process of natural birth. Whenever I was having a moment where I felt hopeless, or where I started to panic, she was there to reassure me. She took my lead and gave me exactly what I needed and nothing more. For me, that mostly came in the form of holding my hand and whispering quietly about how my body was meant to do this.

My doula and Dan helped me labor into the evening. Whenever I would tense my body, the pain would intensify. So, I did everything in my power to stay focused on relaxation. I swayed while holding onto Dan for support. I used the birthing sling to have gravity lend a hand. I sat on the toilet to open my cervix up.

While in transition, I did start to feel that I couldn't go on. We decided to break my water when I was at 9 cm. It was refreshing to make the decision on my own without feeling pressure. It worked well and the baby came down quickly.

For my previous two births, I was given so many instructions along the way that I didn't feel in charge of my own body. This time, I was the only one in charge. Momentarily, this made me feel anxious. "Why wasn't anyone telling me what to do?" I asked myself. But, pretty quickly, my body took over. It did what it was meant to do.

I got back into the tub, and within a short amount of time, I felt myself pushing. I quickly moved her down through the birth canal, and before I knew it, her head was out. The rest of her body proved to be more difficult. They kept telling me to push harder. Finally, Paula said I needed to get out of the tub. In my mind I was thinking, "Get out of the tub with a head between my legs? Are you kidding me??" But you do what you have to do for your baby. So, with help from everyone, I got out of the tub and went to all fours on the floor. Taking the runners pose, Paula told me to keep pushing. I knew that Paula knew exactly what she was doing and that I was in the best possible position for my baby to be born. Paula reached in and grabbed Ana under the armpit and wiggled her out. She was here! They coaxed her to start breathing and Dan handed her through my legs and up to my chest.

Analia Lynn was born at 10:40 p.m., after about eight hours of labor and 10-15 minutes of pushing. She weighed 9 lbs., 11.5 oz.

After getting settled, we took time to get to know one another. Paula sat at the end of the bed and digested the whole experience with me. It felt surreal. It was what I had always wanted. It was definitely intense, but I felt on top of the world. I was proud of myself and proud of my baby.

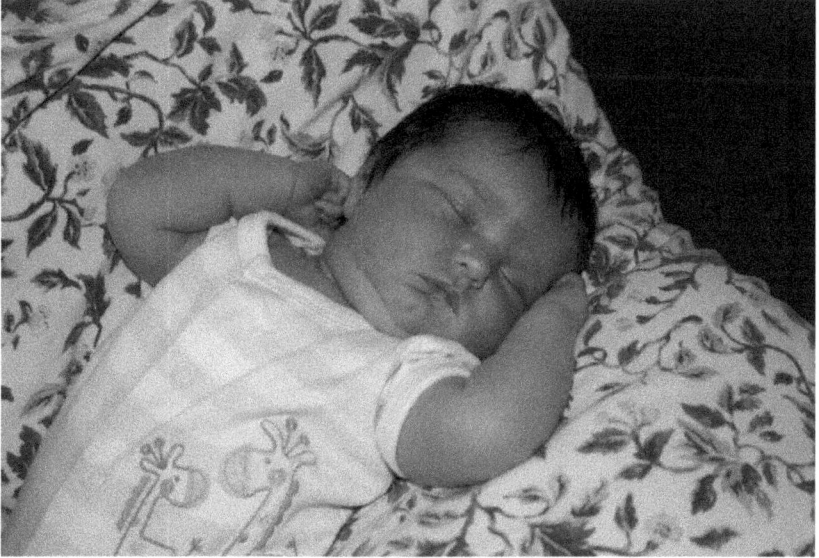

Analia

Part II

**Preparing For
Your Natural Birth**

11

Understanding What Happens During Labor

One way to face labor with confidence is by understanding the process. Labor is divided into three stages. During the first stage of labor, the mother needs to work her relaxation plan to stay calm, while her uterus contracts to move the baby down and the cervix opens. These rushes during the first stage gradually become more intense and closer together with time. This stage can be rather lengthy, especially for first time mothers. It is important during this stage to get rest while you can, in between your rushes, keep hydrated and nourished, and check in with your midwife or doctor. Walking, stretching, and remaining upright as much as possible will help the baby move down. During this first stage, your cervix begins to thin out; this process is called effacement. While it thins, your cervix will also begin to dilate. Practicing open throat vocalizations will also help the process along. During this stage your water is likely to break if it has not already. Sometimes, the bag of waters does not break on its own. If your water does break, you may see all or part of your mucus plug come out, and once this occurs, you may bleed a little. This first stage "usually lasts about fifteen hours for a first baby, and less than that if the mother already had a baby" (Gaskin, 1990, p. 336). Still, it is entirely possible for this stage to last 24 hours. That being said, some women have completed this stage in less than one hour. It is possible. Stay calm and mindful of your birth plan. Keep the atmosphere light. Cuddle with a loved one if you can. Try to rest in between your rushes and move freely, letting gravity help you—the challenge lies ahead.

The second stage of labor begins when you are fully dilated and ends when your baby is born. This stage is often the most intense, but it is also relatively short. During this stage, the baby's head will descend as the uterus pushes the baby downward. You may begin to feel a bit out of control as the intensity takes over. Your belly might shudder, and you might find yourself making movements and sounds you did not anticipate. Go with it. This second stage can last a few minutes to a few hours. Remain active in your labor, repeat positive birthing mantras, and keep breathing—your baby will soon be born!

During the third and final stage of labor, the uterus will continue to contract, and you will birth the placenta. This birth is far less strenuous than the birth of your baby. You might hardly even realize it is taking place as you hold and admire your newborn child.

Labor and delivery can be very intense at times, but the hard work has a phenomenal reward. If you are feeling tired and the rushes are rocking your world, remind yourself that it will all soon be over. Many women are surprised to find true relief after the birth. You are in for a real treat when those rushes cease and the natural endorphins kick in. Happy baby love time!

12

Preparing for the Challenge

One of the misconceptions of "gentle" birth is that the experience will be easygoing for the mother. If she is in the ideal environment, surrounded by loving, supportive people, the laboring mother will be able to peacefully push the blissful infant into the world without stress or strain. Birthing, however, is a rigorous event, and while you may have all the essential elements in place to make the event as pleasant as possible, you must prepare yourself for the greatest physical and mental feat of your life.

The birthing process presents an unusual sort of physical contradiction for a mother. You will need to *take control* and yet *let go* simultaneously. Sound confusing? By taking control, I mean you will need to commit to the physical and mental challenge that is birthing. You should learn all you can about the physical and hormonal processes the body undergoes during labor and birth, so you can assist, not hinder, the course of action. In the exceptional book, *Birthing From Within*, Pam England, CNM, MA, and Rob Horowitz, PhD, discuss the essential need for mothers to "prepare to face the rigors of 'battling with nature' without fleeing the battle field when the going gets tough" (p.128). And in most cases, it will get tough. Labor is rough stuff. Most women describe the pain of labor to be the most intense they have experienced in their lives. Understanding the "physiological fact that pain is an essential component of a normal labor, that it is necessary for the release of hormones that control the progress of labor" (Wagner, 2006, p.53) will help a woman preparing for her birth to put that pain in perspective. If there ever was a "good pain," this is it! Embrace the pain, roll with it, breath through it, be open to it, and you will get through it.

There may come a time you will doubt your ability to press on with your drug-free birth plan. So, you need to prepare yourself for these doubts, and when they creep up, remind yourself with every contraction that you are that much closer to meeting your baby. You are that much closer to resting.

"Some women who romanticize labor and birth may struggle to trust their bodies and their babies, fighting the surrendering one must have to let go. They need to understand that they do not have control, but will always have choices: choices about how to respond to their labor. Believe in yourself—trust your body and spiritual intuitiveness."
—Catherine Mascari, CNM

Morning Star Women's Health
& Birth Center

When the baby is born, the pain of the rushes will end, you will be able to rest, and you will be experiencing the greatest natural high known to womankind. I wish I could bottle the feeling!

How do you prepare for this kind of unknown physical and mental challenge? Education! Read as many positive natural birth stories as you can before your due date. From these stories, you will learn numerous tricks and techniques to get you through the rigors of labor and delivery. You will also gain the confidence of knowing that women from all over the world have faced the same kinds of fears and challenges of birthing naturally and succeeded. Remind yourself that you have incredible strength and you were born for this challenge. As you prepare for your labor and birth, make a pledge to yourself and your baby to give it your all.

Consider Hiring a Doula

Birth is likely the most physically and mentally challenging event a woman will ever experience. Having continuous, positive support will profoundly affect a woman's birth experience. Doulas can provide this service. Believing in each woman's strength, a doula offers up her wisdom, shares her experience, and bestows her time and patience to help ensure a positive birth experience for mother and baby.

According to The Doulas of North America (DONA) International, the word "doula" originated in ancient Greece and meant "a woman who serves." While, at the time, the word could denote any female servant, it came to mean the favorite female servant who would assist the women of the house during childbirth. Today, doulas do more than just serve. Today, doulas guide, nurture, and support. There are two main categories of modern doulas: birth or labor doulas and postpartum doulas. Birth or Labor Doulas are trained professionals who provide continuous physical, emotional, and informational support to the mother before, during, and just after birth. Postpartum Doulas provide emotional and hands-on support directly after the birth of the baby, offering advice to the new mother and providing assistance with light household duties. Many doulas offer both labor and postpartum support, guiding mothers through the passage of birth and the transition to motherhood.

While there are several excellent pathways for doula training available internationally, it is important to realize that skill sets and experience varies, and you need to be an educated consumer when searching for the right labor companion for your birth. The term doula could mean a trained and certified professional, but it could also refer to any friend, family member, or veritable stranger who is willing to provide you with continuous focused support during and/or after the birth of your baby. If you are only interested in hiring a doula with experience and training, be sure to check for credentials.

The main purpose of a birth doula is to help reduce stress during labor and to help keep the mother focused and calm. While fathers and other family members may offer encouragement and support to foster a favorable birthing environment, a trained doula will be able to supplement that support with additional reassurance and skills. The doula may act as a guide to both the laboring mother and her partner. Doulas can also serve as advocates for the mother's wishes and help the family and hospital staff better understand each other's roles and needs. The continuous support offered by a doula is oftentimes the essential ingredient to a positive birthing experience.

"Doula support is very helpful if you wish to avoid pain medication during labor. In our birth culture, epidurals are ubiquitous. Each mom has to think about epidurals before birth and come to her own conclusions. I did a survey of birthing mothers' opinions of their pain medication-free births. These women were from all parts of the country. They were different ages and many of them had several births, some of them with pain medication, some without. I asked many questions in the survey, but the most fascinating one was when I asked the moms if they were glad that they had a birth without pain medications. One hundred percent of the mothers said they were glad they had a pain medication-free birth. They were proud of their accomplishment. It was an accomplishment no one could take away. I was so impressed that every mother surveyed said she was glad!"—Teresa F. Bailey

"Heart & Hands" Doula Service

More than a dozen random trials conducted in different countries with different populations "consistently found benefits" (Goer, 1999) from the presence of doulas during birth. These trails have shown:

> ...the continuous presence of a caring, experienced woman can reduce the length of labor, the use of pain medication, the need for intravenous oxytocin (trade name: Pitocin or "Pit") to stimulate stronger contractions, the likelihood of having an episiotomy (snipping or cutting the vaginal opening), the percentage of instrumental vaginal deliveries, and the C-section

rate…women who have a doula experience less pain and anxiety in labor, express greater satisfaction with the labor, feel they coped better, have a heightened appreciation of their bodies' strength and performance and themselves as women, breastfeed longer, and experience less difficulty in mothering (Goer, 1999, p. 179).

As you have read in many of the birth stories in this book, laboring moms are often immeasurably grateful for the dedicated assistance their doulas provided during the rigors of labor, and they never forget the invaluable support their doulas provided in the hours and days after the birth, allowing the new moms to rest and connect with their new babies.

13

Relaxing During Labor

Every woman is unique and will find different ways to relax during labor. Sometimes just having the right people around during your birth allows you to remain relaxed. Being in a clean and comfortable setting will also help. There are many elements to consider. Time and again, the women who contributed their stories to this book noted water as one of their best relaxation tools. Soaking in the tub, swimming in a warm pool, and relaxing under a shower can help release tension and help you stay loose and unclenched. In advance of your birth, consider the elements that make you feel better when you are uncomfortable and add the following to your birth day bag of tricks if they are not yet there:

- Candlelight
- Dim lighting
- Aromatherapy
- Guided meditation
- HypnoBirthing CDs
- Yoga
- Your favorite peaceful music
- A focal point (a peaceful picture, a small figurine)
- Acupressure
- Deep breathing
- Rhythmic movements
- Soft pillows to straddle

- A hot water bottle
  - Massage
  - Cuddling
  - Humor

14

Turn to the Experts
—Read Ina May!

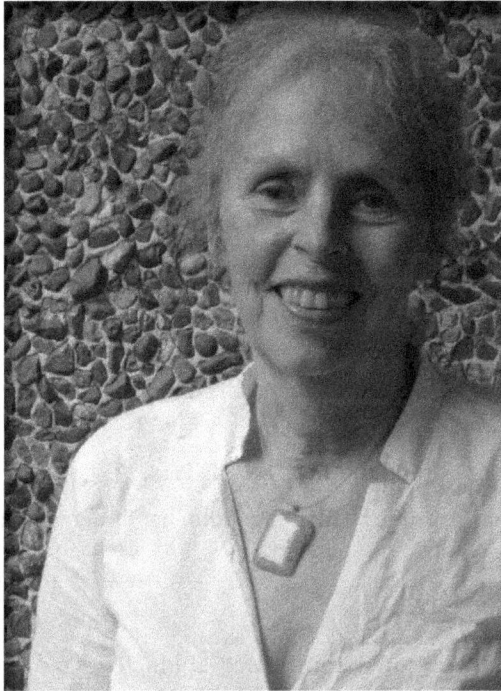

Ina May Gaskin
Photo courtesy of Stephen Gaskin

There is a terrific list of recommended reading in the back of this book, but if you have limited reading time, there might not be a more useful way to prepare for natural childbirth than reading the works of Ina May Gaskin. Gaskin is widely regarded as the leading midwife in the United States. Gaskin's personal experience as a certified professional midwife and extensive research make her plain-spoken explanation of the laboring and birthing process both commanding and accessible to all interested in learning how to avoid interventive, medicalized birth. Many of the birth story contributors in this book make mention of one or more of Ina May's books as being instrumental in building their confidence and essential to their natural birthing success.

Gaskin has written extensively on the subject of women's reproductive health and the birthing process. Her books *Spiritual Midwifery*, *Ina May's Guide to Childbirth*, *Ina May's Guide to Breastfeeding* and *Birth Matters* have helped millions of birthing mothers understand and appreciate what their bodies are capable of. Ina May Gaskin is not a household name in this country, but it should be. Ina May has earned respect and admiration from parents, midwives, doulas, obstetricians, and birth educators all over the world in part due to her impressive personal record of low birth morbidity and mortality and the exceptionally low rate of medical interventions needed at births she has attended.

For the full breadth of Ina May's wisdom, one must read her books, but a brief explanation of some of Gaskin's key ideas will give an expectant woman a good place to begin. Ina May recommends that women and their birth attendants (partners, doulas, midwives) keep in mind four basic concepts that will improve natural birthing outcomes:

1. Understand the Sphincter Law.
2. Keep Oxytocin and Beta-endorphin levels as high as possible and adrenaline levels low.
3. Let the birthing mother take the lead.
4. Let the birthing mother tap into her inner animal—"Trust her monkey self."

The Sphincter Law

Ina May Gaskin invented the name "Sphincter Law" to help women understand the physiognomy of the birthing process. The concept is relatively simple. In her *Guidebook to Childbirth*, Ina May explains that "sphincters are circular muscle groups that ordinarily remain contracted, so the openings of certain organs are held closed until something needs to pass through" (2003, p.170). Most of us have never considered the workings of the sphincter muscles in our bodies. However, understanding them will allow you to help the cervical and vaginal sphincters do their jobs. Ina May explains, "sphincters cannot be opened at will and do not respond well to commands (such as "Push!" or "Relax!") (p. 170). It is important to understand that the sphincters may suddenly close if the birthing mother becomes "upset, frightened, humiliated, or self-conscious" (p. 170). Maintaining a calm and peaceful birthing environment without interruptions will help the sphincters do their work. One of the most amazing considerations of the Sphincter Law is that there is a direct correlation between the relaxation of the mouth and jaw and the ability of the cervix and vagina to open. Take a moment from your reading, look up at the ceiling, and open your mouth wide. Did you feel a loosening down below? See!

I put my newfound understanding of the Sphincter Law into action during my second labor and experienced amazing results. I peacefully labored through the night alone while my husband and daughter slept. Throughout the process I kept my jaw relaxed, throat open, and opened up my hands and fingers as wide as I could make them go, determined to do the opposite of what I did during my first labor, which was roll up into a little ball, furrow my brow, and clench my fists. I dilated steadily and was ready to push when I arrived at the birth center. It really worked!

Of course, what worked for me, won't necessarily work for you. The goal is to find a position that feels comfortable and a rhythm that lets your body work that baby out. But do not forget the Sphincter Law—I am sure it will help you in one way or another!

Encourage the Love Hormones

During labor and birth, a woman's hormones will experience some of the most dramatic shifts of a lifetime. Finding ways of naturally increasing your endorphins will help facilitate a quicker, less painful, more pleasurable birthing experience. Decreasing the levels of adrenaline, which can possibly make a birthing mother labor longer and experience increased feelings of fear and doubt will also help labor progress. You can encourage your endorphins to take a lead role in your labor by communicating with your birth supporters openly and practicing your relaxation techniques. If you feel like you are getting into a rut, make a change. Change position, tell a joke, and move on.

Take The Lead and Let Your Wishes Be Known

A mother-centered birth is a beautiful event. Do not be afraid to let your supporters know exactly what your birthing wishes are and how they might play a part.

Perhaps you'd like to try leg shaking to ease tough contractions. Don't be too shy to ask. They are there to assist you.

When my rushes became so intense that they were literally shaking me, I asked my husband to hug me very tightly. I leaned into his embrace and let him take on part of the intensity for me. I surrendered to the experience and knew I needed more support. I asked him to hold me tighter for the next one, and like this we slowly made our way out to our car to leave for the birth center. Asking for help is easier for some women than others. While some women feel fine laboring and birthing without much assistance, it is important to surround yourself with people you know will be able to support you whatever needs arise during your birthing experience. If you do not feel your spouse or partner will be able to fully carry out the means necessary to support you through this experience, I strongly recommend you reach out for additional support. Consider hiring a doula.

Finally, an Opportunity to Moo!

Ina May has seen that women who allow themselves to move and make sounds instinctually, without allowing their inhibitions to get in the way, will progress through the stages of birth very successfully. You need to loosen up as much as possible and tap into your inner ape, as Ina May suggests. Let the primal mammalian instincts guide you. Many woman claim low moaning, like a cow, works wonders for staying loose and opening the cervix. I gave it a try, but found making cow sounds to be uncomfortable. I needed a higher octave. Whatever sound you make to find comfort, whatever strange position you get into … it's all good.

The birthing body will want to move in a certain way. It will want to make strange noises. Your mind might be saying something like, "Oh, gosh … I probably look like a maniac right now." But listen, sister, you are not at a cocktail party. You've got to let that kind of thinking pass quickly. I spent most of my time riding up and down on the waves of my rushes, with my tongue fully extended like Gene Simmons from KISS. Do you think that looked normal? But it felt right. And I dilated quickly!

During the entire fifteen minutes I was in the birthing tub, my tongue was firmly pressed over my upper lip, while I gripped my inner thighs for leverage. I couldn't help the tongue, it went where it needed to for me, and my body crunched up instinctively to help shorten the birth canal. I did not make much noise during the pushing stage, but blew out air when I needed to. I see now that my "inner animal" was an armadillo—tough yet quiet.

Be courageous, be brave, and trust in your body to lead the way. Like a Patronus in the Harry Potter stories, your inner animal might not reveal itself to you until you need it most. Just be open to its arrival and it will be there to help you!

15

Other Essential Techniques and Tools for Managing the Intensity of Labor

As labor grows increasingly intense, you may need to try one or all of the following measures to help you reach your goal. Your well-trained midwife and doula will have other creative suggestions to add to this list.

Mantras Work

A mantra is a word or short phrase that you can repeat to help keep yourself concentrating on your goal. A mantra can be a powerful tool to help you stay focused and positive during your pregnancy and labor. Many of the moms, birth companions, and attendants I spoke with while writing this book shared their favorite birthing mantras with me. Feel free to borrow one of these or use them as inspiration to create your own.

Move Down, Open Up

I love you, I love you, I love you

I am strong

I can do this

We can do this

Peace

Labor ends

I am a warrior woman

Sterile Water Injections

Sterile Water Injections are simple. Either a midwife or a nurse will inject sterile water into the dimples on the small of your back. The water creates a stinging sensation, which activates the release of endorphins, easing the pain in that area. This technique can be especially helpful for women experiencing painful back labor. (Not all hospitals or birth centers regularly offer this option, so if this sounds like something you may want available, be sure to check well in advance of your labor.) Not keen on needles? Try acupressure.

Acupressure

Acupressure, also called shiatsu, does not involve needles. Instead, fingers apply pressure to various pain-controlling points on the body to relieve pain. You can get your partner some acupressure lessons before the birth as a present, refer to books for guidance, or hire an acupressure specialist to attend your birth.

Hydrotherapy

You may be surprised how effective warm water is for relieving pain. Laboring in a tub helps take some of the pressure off your body, letting your body float in the water and displacing a lot of your weight. You may also want to try focusing the shower stream on the small of your back to help relieve pain and pressure you are feeling in that area. Be forewarned that the tub is the perfect place for many laboring women, but might not feel good for you. It is certainly worth giving it a try!

Shake It Off!

If you are the kind of person who is comfortable accepting hands-on help during labor, let your birth supporters give you a vigorous shakedown when labor starts to feel really intense. If you are looking for something to break the monotony of the rushes, ask your midwife, doula, husband, sister, or whoever you've got to grab a hold of your hips and thighs and shake you. That's right, shake you! Let that mama bootie move! The exact technique can vary. Grasping the upper thigh with two hands and shaking it rapidly forward and backward with the same motion one would use to warm up cold hands is a good technique to start with. Then have your support team try different spots, moving around your buttocks, hips, and thighs. This technique often eases pain and draws your attention away from the heat of the rushes and outwards. Most women who have tried this technique find the shaking itself feels really great. Again, it is worth a try! Just be sure to have a firm hold on the back of a stable chair, couch, or banister—anything to keep you from losing your balance.

The Power of the Mind/Body Connection: The Importance of Tying Up Loose Ends

One story that really hit home for me when I was preparing for my natural birth was one I read in *Ina May's Guide to Childbirth* (pp. 133-135). It described a woman who was having a difficult time progressing through labor. She was in pain and not able to relax in any way. The midwife who was attending became aware of tension between the laboring mom and her husband, and decided to speak up. By intervening, the midwife was able to get the woman to talk through a major issue she was having with her husband, and put it to rest. Almost immediately after this breakthrough, the woman began to dilate rapidly and her baby was soon born.

Be aware of the incredible power of the mind/body connection during birth. Our negative emotions, grudges, fears, and doubts can all be roadblocks to progress during labor. Make it a point to clear your head of all pending emotional baggage before the birth. Do your best to let go of any issue that is creating negativity in your mind. Taking the time to walk yourself through your issues before the birth will help you prepare in a mindful way. Some of your emotional baggage may seem trifling or may seem to have no direct connection to your birth, but if it is taking up space in the corners of your mind, it will do you good to put it to rest. Going into your birth feeling emotionally fresh and confident will help you prepare for the challenges of birthing and motherhood.

16

"Natural" Ways to Stimulate Labor

I remember asking my midwife if she could recommend any natural means for inducing or stimulating labor. She gave me a sort of sideways look. I knew her well enough to realize this meant, "Why?"

Let's face it. Sometimes, when one's due date is close or maybe has passed, the baby is low, the ankles are swollen, and it has become so hard to even stand up, the idea of speeding things up seems very appealing. But most midwives will tell you, it is best to hang in and let your body decide when the time is right. Spontaneous labor, in most cases, is the safest. While you may feel anxious to speed things up, you will be doing yourself and your baby a favor by shifting that anxious energy to a more productive activity— resting.

Depending upon the style of birth you have planned, you might find yourself wanting to try some sort of "natural" form of induction in order to avoid a medical induction. There are various ways to induce labor without pharmaceuticals, each varying in risk.

Nipple Stimulation

Nipple stimulation causes the release of oxytocin, which sometimes initiates or strengthens labor rushes. You can do this yourself manually or by using a breast pump. You can also invite your partner to help. They may even be overjoyed to participate!

Sexual Intercourse

There is a compound in semen that has been found to help ripen the cervix by releasing oxytocin. To avoid possible infection, never engage in sexual intercourse if your water has broken.

Castor Oil

Believed to stimulate the digestive system, castor oil is sometimes effective in stimulating labor. Be forewarned—castor oil can cause diarrhea. Still, you might have diarrhea during labor either way.

Stripping or Sweeping of the Membranes

Your midwife or doctor will insert a finger during a vaginal exam and lift the amniotic sac off your cervix. This procedure is often enough to stimulate rushes and release prostaglandins to ripen the cervix, but can also lead to inadvertent rupturing of the membranes.

Rupturing the Membranes

Also called amniotomy, during this procedure your midwife or doctor will insert an amniohook into the vagina and gently snag the membranes, breaking the bag of waters. Studies have shown that early amniotomy increases the risk of maternal infection (Goer, 1999, p.100). While an amniotomy may reduce your need to be medically induced, it also increases the risk of abnormal fetal heart rate patterns and increases your likeliness of having a C-section (Goer, 1999, p. 103). To further educate yourself about this and other important choices, I highly recommend you read *The Thinking Woman's Guide to a Better Birth* by Henci Goer.

About Medical Inductions

Medical inductions are on the rise for a myriad of reasons, primarily convenience. Whatever your reason for considering inducing your labor, be forewarned "induced labors are much more painful than labors that begin spontaneously, and they lead more often to C-sections as well" (Gaskin, 2011, p. 121). Moreover, medical inductions are not advisable for women who have had previous C-sections or uterine surgery because they bring on such powerful rushes.

If there is a reason for induction, try "natural" measures first before agreeing to a medical induction. Another warning: If you legitimately need a medical induction, be sure to ask your care provider which drug he or she intends to use. Most likely you will be offered intravenous Pitocin, a synthetic form of oxytocin, or a prostaglandin suppository, like Cervidil (dinoprostone), that would be placed into the vagina. Be sure to educate yourself beforehand of the risks of using this drug. It is of utmost importance that you avoid the use of Cytotec (misoprostol) for inductions at all costs. Cytotec is responsible for at least 100 maternal and infant deaths since the 1990s. Furthermore, Cytotec is not FDA-approved for use in pregnant women, nor is it intended for inductions, yet it is still being administered (Gaskin, 2011, p.122). You have the right to know what drugs are being used before they are administered, but will most likely not be told unless you ask. Stand up for your health and the health of your child, and harness the courage to say no when it is needed. Do your homework.

Part III

Natural Birth in the Hospital

17

Birthing Naturally in the Hospital

Hospitals are still the places the majority of American women are choosing to birth. Despite the growing availability of birth centers and home midwives, many pregnant women still believe hospitals are their best option, and many do not even investigate other possibilities. Some expectant women choose hospital birth to be close to pain-easing medications, emergency equipment, and those trained to use it. Still others choose hospitals fully intending to birth naturally, feeling at ease with the environment, and aware of the challenges and pressures.

However, women who deeply desire to birth without interventions may experience additional challenges as they labor in a hospital. As their contractions intensify, often are the offerings to dull the sensation with medication. It is easy to lose focus of a natural birth when one is in an environment that defies nature—the lighting is artificial, the smell of disinfectant is laden in the air, machines are humming. It is also more challenging to relax when a steady stream of strangers are marching in and out authoritatively with clipboards and name tags. Being aware of the "normal" every day routine of a labor and delivery ward will allow the natural birthing mother to prepare for these less than natural, less than comforting features and make a plan.

One of the best ways to avoid unnecessary interventions while laboring in a hospital is to have a well-educated spokesperson advocating your desires to the hospital staff. A midwife will be a wonderful advocate, especially one that works regularly with the hospital you choose. A doula is another tremendous support, for she will also be able to help keep you focused and buy you more time to let nature take its course. You do not want to find yourself in the uncomfortable situation of trying to birth your baby naturally, while haggling with the nurses to give you more time to progress without calling in the doctor and pressuring you to accept Pitocin. Have your informed ring of support in place to speak for you, so you can stay in the moment and stay in your zone.

"Stay home! Especially in early labor, if you have no complications, STAY HOME! The less time you are with your care provider, the fewer chances that he/she will want to "do" something to "help" you along." —Catherine Parisi, CNM, MSN

Connecticut Childbirth & Women's Center

If circumstances out of your control require you to be transferred to a hospital, upturning your peaceful birth center or home birth dream, do not despair. While the environment may not be exactly what you had hoped for, the experience does not have to be any less mindful, meaningful, and beautiful. Any "complication" that "risks you out" of birthing at home or in a free-standing birth center will add stress to your labor, but that stress can be overcome if you anticipate it and breath through it. You will need to dig a little deeper to retain focus and remind yourself that women can and do deliver naturally in hospitals every day of the year, and chances are you can, too. No matter where you end up birthing, whether in your home, in a car, or in a birth center, you have to accept that there are certain elements that will always be out of your control no matter how calm or prepared you are.

18

Choosing Interventions Mindfully

Sometimes, despite your best efforts, you and your birth team will decide that a medical intervention is a good choice. Perhaps, your labor is unexpectedly long and intense and you are utterly exhausted—an epidural may help you get a little rest and regain the strength you need to make the final effort to push your baby out. Perhaps, labor has stalled and you and your midwife have tried to talk through any possible psychological roadblocks, and no matter what kind of creative position your midwife puts you in, it does not pick up. You have tried everything: nipple stimulation, walking stairs, the tub, acupressure, bouncing on a ball, and still labor will not progress. There might be a genuine need for intervention. A long list of unexpected possibilities could arise, changing the game plan and necessitating you to abandon your initial intention to birth without drugs. There are valid reasons to apply interventions, and when used appropriately, they can often prevent you from needing a more serious intervention or be truly lifesaving. If you have chosen a birth team that you trust, making the decision to accept an intervention will be easier and less stressful.

Going into labor mindful that complications can arise will make shifting gears and going with the flow much easier and acceptable. In their iconic book *Birthing from Within*, Pam England and Rob Horowitz write, "If labor is abnormal and the benefits of drugs or anesthesia outweigh their risks, welcome them. Accept that you did the best that you could, and stay present and involved in your birth in every way you can. Remember, an epidural doesn't need to stop you from birthing from within" (1998, p. 254). Despite our best effort, we cannot control the universe … still, we do have control over the choices we make and our attitude about those choices.

19

The Beautiful Hospital Birth of My Big Baby Luke: It is Possible!

By Nancy Kelly

Not once before my pregnancy had I considered how I would birth my baby. I guess I just assumed women did this all the time, and I didn't really need to worry too much about it. The midwives would tell me what to do, I would go to the hospital, follow directions, and have my baby. I thought it was as simple as that. Yet, halfway through my pregnancy, I realized, wow, I actually have to push this baby out of me, and it suddenly seemed extremely overwhelming. I started my exploration of birthing choices by reading the book *Easy Labor* by William Camann, MD, and Kathryn Alexander, MA, which offered details on all options for laboring women.

As I read the book, I felt especially connected to the sections on natural birthing choices. When I read about using doulas and hypnosis to support a natural birth, I began researching both options, and within a week, I had found both an amazing doula (who is still my friend today) and a fantastic hypnosis program for birth called Hypnobabies. I worked with both to learn about natural birth and deep relaxation to make my birthing time wonderful, and in the weeks that passed, I began to believe that my baby's birth would be a peaceful and joyous experience for all of us.

Weeks and months passed. I was the type of expectant mom who assumed that my baby would come any time after 37 weeks. That's considered full-term, after all, and I had waited so long already. Surely my baby wouldn't keep me waiting too much longer...

Well, I would be in for nearly another five weeks of pregnancy! I kept moving ahead with my hypnosis practice, as I anxiously awaited my baby's arrival.

It was early March, and I had lived by that February 21st due date for nearly ten months, which felt like a lifetime to me as a first-time mom. As each day passed, I wondered if he would ever come at all. Then, on a Monday morning, at my 41–week appointment, the midwife used the dreaded word—induction—and I became even more determined to meet my baby. Because I was working with a large city hospital midwife practice, I knew that I needed to have my baby by 42 weeks if I wanted to avoid medical induction. All of the things I had been doing—evening primrose oil, walking, spicy foods, sex—had not brought the baby so far; therefore, I immediately called my doula, asking about some of the more serious natural induction methods, and was on my way to a special prenatal chiropractor on Tuesday and an acupuncturist on Wednesday.

In the early hours of the morning on Thursday, my birthing waves began, and I was blessing that chiropractor and acupuncturist! After using the bathroom, I gently woke my husband to tell him I thought we would meet our baby soon. We were both so excited we couldn't sleep anymore. I stayed in bed to focus on my waves, which were coming every 15 or 20 minutes, and he went downstairs to clean up a bit and make some food. The morning passed peacefully, with me listening to my Hypnobabies tracks, eating a bit, and sleeping on and off. By early afternoon, we decided to call my parents and sister to let them know the time was upon us. We had already planned for my mom and sister to attend the birth with us.

By mid-afternoon, my birthing waves became more intense, and my family arrived at our home. I definitely needed to focus on each wave as it came. I spent a few hours leaning on my birth ball, but time was not moving normally for me. An hour would pass in what seemed like 15 minutes. I attribute this to my deep relaxation. As each wave would come over me, I would let every abdominal muscle relax, and I would think to myself, "let your body do the work... don't fight this...." Those thoughts kept me calm and in control.

Evening came, and my family had dinner. I tried to eat some, but I was a bit nauseous and just couldn't keep anything down at that point. Again, the hours passed by so quickly that before I knew it, it was time for bed again. I decided I would try to sleep, but I quickly realized my bed was not a good place for me. I wasn't at all comfortable lying on my bed in any position. This was the first time I felt frustrated. I was so tired, I really wanted to rest my head and body, but I knew I would have to keep vigil on this night. I spent the night alternating between leaning on the birth ball, rocking in the rocking chair, bouncing on the ball, and leaning on the bed. My sister went home to sleep, and my husband and mom kept me going through the night. They each got a few hours of sleep, alternating keeping me company during the long nighttime hours.

I don't know if my attitude changed or the waves became more intense, but the middle of the night was the longest and hardest part of my birthing time. I couldn't help but think of the rest of the world sleeping and resting, and I felt jealous. Thank goodness I had my mom and husband with me! They helped me adjust my attitude during those hours. When I doubted my ability to get through it, my husband told me to get through five more waves, then see how I felt. I was talking about going to the hospital, but I was nervous that if I got there, and I found out I wasn't as far along as I had hoped, I would request pain medication. Both my mom and husband found words that helped me. They left the decision in my hands, but supported me with inspiring words and reminders that I was doing really well. We called my doula to let her know what was going on, and she had us check in with her every hour or so until about 5:00 a.m., when she came to our house to join us.

The light of day was such a beautiful sight! With the sun, came the arrival of my sister and my doula. My waves continued to be intense, but with the pleasure of company and my doula's suggestions for different positions (including climbing the stairs over and over), time began to pass quickly again. By about 9:00 a.m., we decided to begin our move to the hospital.

Once we arrived, I was checked, and found to be about 6 centimeters dilated. I knew it was only a number, but I was pretty happy with it, as it seemed I was at least moving in the right direction. The nurses thought I was dehydrated from the frequent vomiting, and since I really couldn't keep even liquids down, I allowed an IV and one bag of fluids. After that, the IV stayed in place on my arm, but was not hooked to any medications.

I was transferred to one of the low-intervention rooms and was assigned to a natural birth-friendly nurse. She encouraged me to take small sips and bites here and there, which was a surprise, as I believe the hospital has a "nothing by mouth" policy. It was nice to know that my nurse was more concerned about me and my baby than hospital policies.

Unfortunately, with the excitement of the move to the hospital, my waves slowed and I began to feel discouraged. My doula suggested a shower to get things moving again. A few hours into our hospital stay, the waves picked up again, and I could feel some moderate progression. I had wanted an intervention-free birth, but when the midwife checked me, and found me to be less than 8 centimeters dilated, she offered to break my bag of waters in the hopes of moving things along. After over 35 hours of birthing waves, I was eager to pick up the pace, and in that moment, having her break my bag of waters seemed like a reasonable intervention. Within 30 minutes, my waves picked up again, and I was in transition.

My amazing doula recommended waiting to use the Jacuzzi for this time in my birthing. I am glad she did, as it was the most intense part of the birth, and the water helped me stay relaxed and focused.

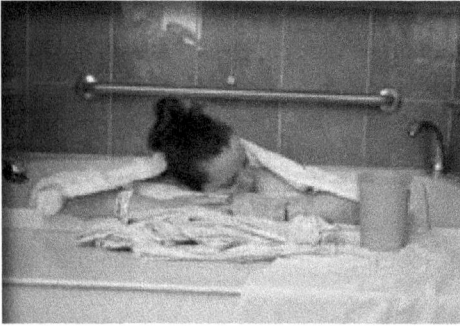

Nancy laboring in the Jacuzzi tub

In our birthing classes, I had learned that many women experience a break in contractions after transition, so I kept asking my doula over and over, "When is that break I'm supposed to have?" She never gave a straight answer, but I guess she didn't want to get my hopes up. I never did get that break!

After the tub, my doula asked me what my body was telling me to do. I didn't know what she meant, so I asked her to be more specific. She asked if it felt like I should push. I didn't have that overwhelming feeling to push that many women have described, so I just gave it a try. For me, it was strange, because I felt like I didn't know what I was doing. I asked for guidance on how to push, and after a few tries, I got the hang of it. In hindsight, I wonder if perhaps I wasn't ready to push, but in that moment, I just wanted to be at the next stage, getting closer to meeting my baby.

I pushed on all fours and I pushed on the birth stool; I pushed on the toilet and the birth chair; I pushed leaning on the birth ball. I pushed on the bed and the floor. I pushed all over that room! My new nurse came on duty, and immediately, we could tell she was very experienced, with a no-nonsense attitude. To be honest, I envisioned the pushing stage to be quick, with me in any position except flat on my back, and I certainly couldn't imagine myself going red in the face during each push. Yet, after three hours of pushing, when the new midwife-on-duty came by to see me, and she didn't like my progress, our nurse suggested I try pushing on my side and back. Because I did not want an assisted delivery, and I could hear that threat in my midwife's voice, I did as my nurse suggested. To my surprise, it was the most comfortable pushing position for me. I truly believe that having everyone see my progress and tell me what they saw, encouraged me to keep going. I had a goal in sight. In fact, I quite literally had my goal in sight, as my sister held a mirror for me to see my baby's head emerging during every push. It was an amazing vision! My nurse encouraged me to touch my baby's head and feel his hair! Wow, with him still inside me, I was able to see and touch him, finally!

Our nurse also gave my husband a job; he used the olive oil we brought with us to manually lubricate the whole area as my baby was coming closer and closer. This was such a great way to keep my husband involved, as well as to prevent injury for me. Even though some men might say no-thank-you to such a duty, my husband took on the role like a champ, and I think he was grateful to have a star role in the birth. I credit him and that bottle of olive oil with keeping my perineum in tact after delivering a big baby.

Time was not passing as usual for me once again. I had no idea how long I had been pushing, or even how long I'd been at the hospital or in labor. All I knew is that as my baby's head emerged a little more each time, I was that much closer to meeting him. The nurse made the call to the midwife that it was time to come back, but she was with another mom at that time, so the resident doctor came to us. After all those months of booking my prenatal appointments with different midwives, so I would have met them all by the time of the birth, here I was, pushing my baby out into the hands of someone I had never met. I was only slightly disappointed by this, because in hindsight, I realize the resident actually had more faith in me than the midwife did. She never once suggested or hinted at any assisting interventions, whereas the midwife was ready to pull out the vacuum.

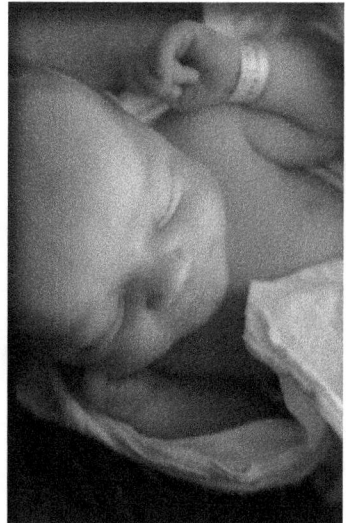

With the doctor dressed and ready for our baby, I gave a few more pushes, and his head was out! Then, with the next push, his shoulders were out. The room grew noisy with excitement. Before the next push, the doctor asked me to reach down, and as I pushed with my belly, I pulled my baby out with my hands. It was magical! The nurse helped ease him onto my chest, where he took his first breath andhis very loud first cry. Luke was born. He was here, finally, after nearly 42 weeks of pregnancy, and 42 hours of labor.

Smiling baby Luke

Luke was 9 lbs, 10 oz, and 21.5 inches long. His head circumference was off the charts. He was declared a "big boy" by our nurse, even before he was weighed. However, there was no number on a scale that would make him anything other than my precious little baby to me.

I was not tired, as I had been even an hour before. I was high on baby. I was high on oxytocin. Our son stayed on me, skin to skin, for what seemed like hours, even though I know it was only an hour or so. Nursing came pretty naturally to both of us in those first hours of life. Within an hour, I was up around the room with some help, and after a few hours of rest, I was walking around on my own, holding my little guy with me wherever I went. I was pleased to have had a comfortable birth, with no complications for me or baby. I recovered well. I had a healthy body to help give us an amazing start to life with our Luke at home with us.

We became a family on that winter night. It was magical and transformative. I am so glad that we experienced birth as it was meant to be. It was everything I hoped it would be, and I have such wonderful memories of the entire experience.

20

Expecting the Unexpected: The Birth of Elowen Ann

By Sayward Parsons

My second pregnancy began in September of 2010 and progressed smoothly until a midwife's visit around March found the baby's heart rate was around 120. Because it was much lower than the previous Doppler results, the midwife, Cathy Gallagher, sent me across the street to the hospital for a longer non-stress test. I was dehydrated and an ultrasound showed nothing to be concerned about, so they sent me on my way. When subsequent non-stress tests showed a fetal baseline in the 90s, I was sent to high-risk pregnancy specialists and to Yale New Haven to visit a world-renowned fetal cardiologist. When one of the midwives delivered the news that I had risked out of giving birth at the Center and would instead have to deliver my baby at Danbury Hospital, my heart sank. This shook everything I had come to believe about pregnancy and labor: they are completely natural human functions that do not require constant monitoring and incessant worry.

While I had found encouragement from the natural birthing books and the Hypnobirthing philosophy throughout my first easy, normal pregnancy, they had also instilled in me a hypersensitivity to unnecessary interventions. I had loved everything about my first birth experience at the Birth Center, and with my new scenario, I began envisioning worst-case scenarios that included IVs, hospital beds, and a large team of doctors with scalpels hovering outside the doors of the delivery room. I somehow had to find a way to reconcile my fear of a "medicalized" birth with the reality that this pregnancy was indeed more complicated.

I quickly got on board with a hospital birth when I realized it meant that the best possible resources would be available for my baby. There was no evidence that there was anything wrong other than a disturbingly low heart rate, but I knew that even a small chance of an emergency transfer to the hospital once the baby was born could waste valuable time. Yet, I still dreaded a hospital birth. Though a midwife would attend the birth and the midwives assured me we could bring the "spirit of the birth center" to the hospital, I wondered whether the birth of my second child could still be as meaningful and intimate.

Toward the end of my pregnancy, I visited the Birth Center three times a week for non-stress tests, each appointment reminding me of the reasons this pregnancy was not as normal as the first: the puzzlingly low heart rate, the midwives' anxiousness, and the unknown reaction of the hospital staff when I showed up in labor with a baby who had such a low heart rate. My spirits were brought even lower when the midwives talked about induction, a word my natural birthing books had taught me to be wary of. I ultimately decided that I had chosen health care providers who I trusted. I did my research and I questioned everyone, but eventually accepted that if I did not go into labor spontaneously by 41 weeks I would be induced.

On Monday, June 13, the day after my due date, I agreed to an internal exam and membrane sweep. Sarah Najamy, another one of the midwives from the Birth Center, said I was one centimeter dilated and about fifty percent effaced. At Wednesday's appointment, I opted not to be checked, but on Thursday, four days after my expected due date, I began feeling surges. I had had Braxton Hicks contractions since my seventh month of this pregnancy, but I could tell these were different.

After a restless night, I asked my husband to stay home on Friday, wishfully thinking something was going to happen. We went to my midwife appointment on Friday afternoon, and I opted for another membrane sweep. Cathy Parisi found I was three centimeters dilated and 80% effaced; I was slightly comforted that things were progressing. "You've already gotten through 30% of your labor!" Cathy optimistically encouraged. She was the midwife I felt was the least anxious about my baby's heart rate; I hoped I would go into labor during her shift that began the next morning. Cathy suggested I get up Saturday morning, try some castor oil, and see what happened.

I had surges all day Friday and practiced deep breathing with each, but they weren't coming any closer together. I woke up with surges nearly every hour that night. Though they caused cramping and achiness, I was more restless than uncomfortable. Around 6:00 a.m., the surges felt stronger. I had to lean against the kitchen counter and use deep breathing to focus on keeping my body relaxed. I decided to take a spoonful of castor oil and the surges seemed to pick up about an hour later. I labored at home for the next couple of hours, getting on my hands and knees to sway with each, the movement easing some of the pressure. I rocked back and forth on a birthing ball and tried to continue drinking water, though I didn't have an appetite for breakfast.

After an initial 8:00 a.m. call, my husband called Cathy around 10:00 and said the surges were quite strong, though still only about 10 minutes apart. Cathy was especially sensitive to my concerns about the hospital. She offered to meet us at the Birth Center and check me before deciding to go to the hospital.

Cathy found me to be six centimeters dilated and almost completely effaced. She said I had two options. Since I was having a slow and steady labor, I could return home and eventually the surges would get closer together or I could go to the hospital where she would break my water and guessed the baby would be here in a few hours. I couldn't envision another sleepless night, and then trying to have a natural birth. I felt I was coping with the surges effectively, but many more hours of them would have totally exhausted me. I opted for the trip to the hospital.

Cathy broke my water around 11:30. At first, I didn't feel a difference, but about 20 minutes later, the surges started intensifying. I got out of bed, where they had been monitoring the heart rate, to use the bathroom and had three strong surges in just a few minutes. I felt intense pressure inside my abdomen and around my sides. It felt like my body was opening in a way it had not for my first labor. I wanted to labor in the tub because it had worked so well for me the first time, but Cathy was afraid it might slow down the contractions. She encouraged me to stay up and moving for a bit. She asked if I needed counter pressure on my back during the surges, which helped a great deal with their growing intensity. I moved to a birthing ball, leaning on the bed with each surge, taking long, loud breaths—the moaning making it somehow easier. I tried not to fight against each contraction, but it hurt to use them, to relax into them the way the midwife was suggesting. I knew I had to, though, so with my husband's steady encouragement, I used each bit of energy the best I could. I started sweating with each, and then the midwife said I could get into the tub if I wanted, but they did not want me birthing in the tub. Because of the baby's low heart rate, which had remained steady throughout labor, Cathy wanted doctors to have instant access to the baby if necessary.

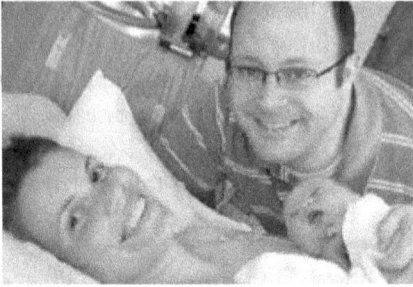

**Sayward with her husband and
Elowen Ann**

I climbed in and had another surge; the water didn't seem to ease the sensation as much as I had remembered. Cathy told me that as soon as I felt the slightest bit of pressure, I had to let them know, so they could immediately get me out of the tub. I told her I had not felt any pressure or urge to push with my first birth, and she said she thought it would be different this time. Sure enough, as I breathed through the next surge, I felt the slightest bit of pressure at the end of it. With the next surge, I felt what I had not expected to and shouted, "I need to push." Somehow, my husband, Cathy, and the student midwife, Miri, helped me out of the tub and into the bed. Cathy directed me to push as hard and for as long as I could with each surge, while a nurse hooked up the fetal heart rate monitor. I pushed with each surge for as long as I could, and when I felt I couldn't push anymore, Cathy and Miri's words encouraged me to try again. From the first push, I felt the baby moving down, an exciting and encouraging feeling I had not had the benefit of the first time around. I pushed for twenty minutes, and it was hard work. At one point, I just wanted to rest and said, "I can't do this." "Yes, you can, you have to," Cathy asserted, and I knew she was right, so I conjured the strength to push again. After only 20 minutes, I birthed the baby's head, and with a final push, the shoulders and body were born. The baby was placed on my chest, and once again my husband was able to announce, "It's a girl."

Elowen Ann was born on June 18, 2011, at 1:39 in the afternoon. The sun shined outside the hospital window, and I was able to hold Elli in my arms as my small tear was stitched up. Her heart rate was still low after the birth, but not a concern since everything else was normal. I was grateful that our baby was a healthy 8 lb 9oz and

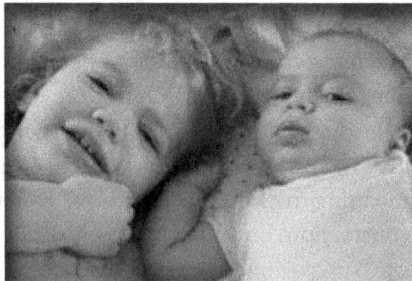

Sisters: Lahja Belle and Elowen Ann

bright eyed. And looking back, I am even grateful for the trials we faced during the pregnancy. I learned a great deal about how each pregnancy brings unique challenges and blessings. I learned that when you have chosen healthcare providers you respect and trust, the difficult decisions become a bit easier to make with their guidance. A commitment to and desire for a natural birth, as well as a supportive partner, created a reserve of strength for me to draw from when labor was at its most challenging. And though both of my daughters' births were unique, they were equally beautiful and equally joyful.

21

Emmett is Born!

By Lori Merhige

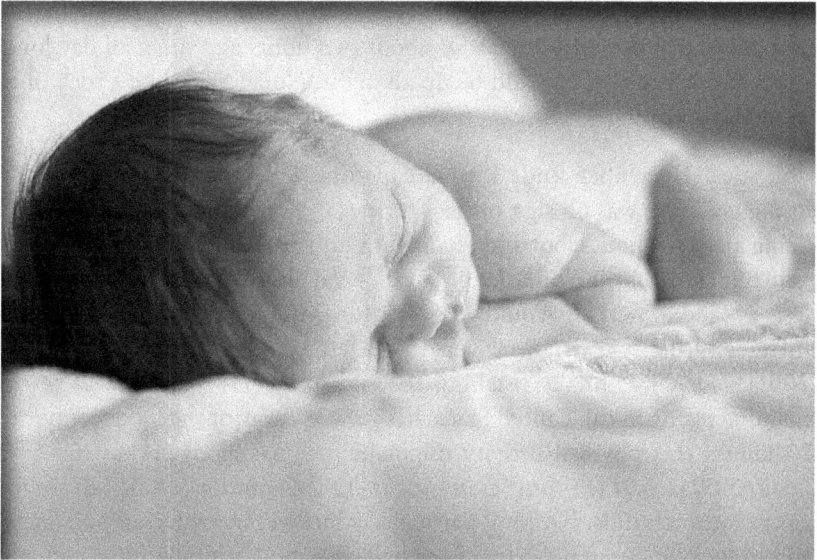

Emmett. Photo courtesy of Elissa A. Betterbid

Because of my diagnosis of gestational diabetes, I went through a ridiculous amount of (over)testing in the last month of my pregnancy. I was at St. Luke's/Roosevelt at least twice a week—ultrasounds on Tuesdays, non-stress tests on Fridays, in addition to appointments with my OB, as well as the Diabetes doctors. Fortunately, the baby measured within the realm of 'normal' and there were no issues for the doctors to report.

I was cleared for delivery in the Birthing Center on a week-to-week basis, beginning at 38 weeks. I was initially given a due date of December 3rd, but my OB moved it up to November 30th around my eighth month. The 30th came and went, and I was a little nervous, as my doc was not going to let me go far past my due date because of the diabetes. At my last appointment with my OB on November 30th, she gave me a rather vigorous pelvic exam to hopefully get things moving. We also made a plan to come back on December 5th for Cervidil. She felt that Cervidil would kick things off, and I'd have my baby by Monday evening (December 6th). If that (and all else) failed, we would have to schedule an induction with Pitocin for Tuesday, December 7th. Yikes!

The good news was that I had been walking around for two to three weeks at 1–2 cm dilated and 80% effaced. The stage was set, but the waiting was the worst! I was okay with the Cervidil plan, but would still be trying everything I could to bring things on naturally. I really wanted labor to start on it's own!

On Wednesday, December 1st, I felt like I had the flu, with fatigue, aches and pains, but no fever. I slept for about two hours at a time, all day long. I was concerned that I would be up all night. Nope. Slept like a rock until Thursday morning.

Thursday, December 2nd, I woke up totally refreshed—good as new. Strangely, there was no sign of the previous day's malaise. I decided to stop being anxious about labor and go on with my life. I ran a few work errands, which included lifting bundles of fabric. I was almost finished handling the last of the orders I would process for my family business in lace manufacturing. I had taken over the daily operations of the company in 2001, and it was finally reaching the end of its 35+ year run, as textile manufacturing in the United States has gone the way of the Dodo. Anyway, I thought this physical activity might help things along. I was right! At about 2:00 p.m., I felt some cramping every few minutes, while I drove my car between errands. Nothing particularly intense, but the cramps came at somewhat regular intervals for about half an hour. I was quietly excited, but didn't get my hopes up.

Things stopped for an hour or so and I returned home. Once I ate a late lunch, the cramps came back! I walked around Weehawken from about 3:40 to 4:50 p.m. Every few minutes I felt slight rushes of pain...finally something was happening! At about 4:30 p.m., I noticed the pain intensified to the point where I had to stop walking and lean on someone's retaining wall until the sensation passed. About 10 minutes later, this happened again. I called Ryan and told him he might want to come home from work a little early...not to rush or panic, but maybe things were starting.

I returned to the apartment thinking I still had lots of time before things got intense. I had plans to cook dinner and make a birthday cake. Ha! Ryan came home and ran out to the supermarket to pick up some ingredients. By the time he returned around 7:00 p.m. or so, I was seriously slowing down. It took an hour to prepare the appetizer, as I had to keep stopping to get on my hands and knees and breathe. This continued with contractions several minutes apart for a while.

I did a lot of vocalization and Ryan was there for each contraction, helping by pressing on my lower back. Somewhere in there, we gave up on cooking, and he called for some takeout. The food arrived, I had a few bites, then went back to my hands and knees, first on a yoga mat on the floor and later on the couch, leaning on pillows and my birth ball. I was rocking, using vocalization, getting back massages, and doing a lot of visualization of me opening. An hour or so later, I got into the hot shower. I was on my hands and knees in the tub with the water hitting my back. That felt great! Then the hot water ran out after only 15 minutes, which sucked. I would have liked to stay in there about an hour longer.

Back on the couch, things seemed to be moving quickly, which was good. I had no concept of time at that point, but somehow knew that labor was progressing. I would ask Ryan every so often what time it was. 9:30 p.m., then 11:00 p.m. ...Ryan was timing contractions and keeping track in a notepad.

Ryan was in touch with our doula, Marin, and eventually she arrived, perhaps between midnight and 1:00 a.m. She got right into it and was great. She immediately sat near me and rocked and massaged my back, while Ryan got things ready for our eventual trip to the hospital. At some point, the tailbone massage stopped feeling good, and I let Marin know that maybe hip compression would feel better. She didn't miss a beat, and even vocalized with me through each contraction. Soon, Marin suggested I try to lie down in bed for a little while, as it was late at night and I needed rest. My legs *were* getting tired from crouching on the sofa. She suggested that I lay there on my side, with lots of pillows and with Ryan next to me, and perhaps I could doze off between contractions.

Things were intense by this point, and at first I thought it was insane to think I could sleep through this. But much to my surprise, I found that each contraction woke me up from a dreamy state. I was actually sleeping in three to four minute intervals! With each contraction, Ryan would squeeze my hand between thumb and index finger, in the hoku acupressure point. It didn't eliminate the pain, but it gave me something else to focus on; and just having him there as a loving and supportive presence was essential.

It was during this time that the contractions took a leap in intensity. My vocalization became a mantra of 'open.' I also used a breathing technique Marin had shown me, where I inhaled up my spine to the top of my head, then exhaled down to 'fill a little cup' in my belly. When I did this nourishing breath, I could feel the baby move! I also silently asked him again and again to please work with me to push himself out and visualized myself opening up. I swear this worked!! Call me crazy, but when I would call on the baby for help, I could feel him and could also feel myself opening!

During this laying down time, contractions were three to four minutes apart. When we hit the 3–1–1 stage (3 minutes apart, 1 minute long, continuously for 1 hour), Ryan called my OB and left a message with her answering service. As we waited for the call back, I continued with the 'open' mantra and the visualization. I began to feel a squishy, liquid-y feel with each contraction, as if a bit of fluid was sloshing out with each wave. I mistakenly attributed this to a bit of mucous or bloody show, which I had been experiencing for a couple of days. It took about an hour for the doctor to call back; it was my OB's partner. She only wanted to talk to me, not Ryan. She asked me if my water had broken, and I said no. She said it sounded like I should make my way to the hospital. After discussing this with Ryan and Marin, we decided to begin to get going, but we'd take our time. It was around this time that I thought I might freak out if I got to the hospital and wasn't *at least* 7 cm dilated. It felt like I was far along—I wanted to be right about that.

It wasn't until I got up to use the bathroom and found myself to be rather wet, that we realized my water had most likely broken, and that the baby's low position was keeping the bulk of it from gushing out. Marin suggested we not take our time and just get going.

I should mention here that I had tested positive for Group B Strep and was required to arrive at the hospital as soon as my water broke, as I was required to spend at least four hours before delivery receiving antibiotics through an IV. Oops! It was also at this point that I realized how very valuable having a knowledgeable doula was—once I got up from the bed, the contractions were not as painful when I was standing, *AND* I was well rested. I felt like I had a second wind!

So, I was loaded into the car, leaning on my luggage with a body pillow over it, on hands and knees in the back seat. Ryan drove, and Marin followed in her car. It was around 3:00 a.m., and it took all of 10 minutes to go through the Lincoln Tunnel and up 10th Avenue to St. Luke's. Marin had advised me as we were getting ready to go that I should try my best to stay 'in it' and not lose focus, or let the distractions of the car ride or the hospital slow things down. I took that to heart and kept my eyes closed most of the time. I was surprised to find, however, that although I was definitely in 'laborland,' I felt very clear headed and able to assess my situation quite well. I guess that's what they mean when they say you should let go and travel 'within,' rather than try to move outside of yourself. I even was able to do a little back-seat driving in between contractions!

I wonder if the guy at the parking garage was freaked out by my bending over to lean on our hospital suitcase in the middle of his parking lot to have a very vocal contraction as soon as I got out of the car? I can say with certainty that I couldn't care less at the time. And that's how it went—a contraction on the sidewalk, one in the emergency room, one in the hallway, where we spared the lone man in the elevator my moaning while we waited for the next one. St. Luke's has those nifty guardrails along the hallways outside of the triage room—very handy when you need to bend over and yell a little bit.

Triage was a little rough. Ryan had to fill out forms as I leaned forward over the waiting room chair, yelling 'ooooopppppeeeennnn,' while Marin spoke softly to me and rocked my hips. There were other people there, and they probably thought I was possessed, but I didn't care at that point. I kept my eyes closed the entire time. Then they took me in by myself. I had to put on a gown and a girdle (seriously?) and pee in a cup, which required me to give myself a pep talk, now that Ryan was not here to hold my hand. I am still somewhat amazed that I was able to deliver a urine sample, but not without leaving a bit of a mess on the bathroom floor. Then they put the monitors on me and laid me down. I immediately understood all that stuff I read about how being immobile and laying on your back brings you closer to needing an epidural. I communicated how much it sucked to the nurse, who did what she could and raised the headrest about six inches. Thanks. Thanks a lot.

There were a lot of questions at that point, and I answered between contractions. They took blood and asked me about three times about my Group B Strep status. There was a delay of what seemed like a while before they put in the IV with the antibiotics. They took my blood and checked my blood sugar. All the while I was squirming and moaning very loudly through the contractions. I could hear other, calmer sounding women in labor talking normally in the other triage stations. Again, it didn't take much for me to not be self-conscious about how loud I was being.

The nurse examined me and said I was 7 cm dilated. Hooray!

Finally, they let Ryan come in to the room. He asked if I needed anything and I asked for water. He had been great with the squirt bottle all night—we had stocked up on Gatorade and coconut water. But the nurse said I couldn't drink water and Ryan and I exchanged a look. We'd have to wait for the doctor's okay, she said. He held my hand and tried not to look frazzled at being in 'the system' at this point.

At last the OB came in (my OB's partner) and I remember thinking she looked different than when I met her in my doctor's office a few weeks ago. I then remembered it was about 4:00 in the morning. She seemed a little frazzled at first, especially when I admitted that I think my water *did* in fact break, probably an hour before I spoke with her on the phone. I can't recall if it was she or the nurse who said, while administering the IV antibiotics, that hopefully it would be more than four more hours before I delivered that baby or else the baby would have to stay in the hospital for 48 hours for observation. I distinctly remember thinking that this was sure as hell NOT going to go on for four more hours if I could help it!

Another pelvic exam by the OB confirmed that yes, I was 7 cm, and yes, my waters did break. With that, a gush of water came out and there was a sudden relief of pressure for about two seconds. Then the contractions took on a new, fuller force. Once the antibiotics were fully administered, it was time to get in the wheelchair and go to the birthing center. As I stood up, water gushed out of me, and I stood there in it in my socks. I actually felt kinda bad for making a mess! The doctor was like, 'Oh, don't worry about it!' It's great to be around people who have seen it all. It was hard to sit down, though. I could feel the baby's head and the pressure was increasing with each minute. I kept my eyes closed and the doctor wheeled me over to the birthing center.

We got to the room, and at this point I was well into transition. The contractions were capped by an intense pressure and urge to push. In fact, I was sort of involuntarily pushing at the end of each contraction. Needless to say, I was LOUD. Marin helped me lean over the bed while the nurse brought a birthing ball. I couldn't even sit on this soft surface—I squatted over it. My legs were shaking; Ryan spotted me as I squatted. I had my moment of self-doubt and said, "I don't think I can do this for much longer." Ryan and Marin were quick with reassurance. They offered the hot tub and I said yes. Ryan filled the tub, which seemed to take forever to fill. I yelled into my pillow with increasing intensity. Finally, the tub was full and I got in. I hate to say it, but at this stage in the game, it wasn't as relieving as I wished it would be. The warm water felt nice, but I was at that integral point where your body is giving you all it can handle. The tub was large and I kind of floated around in there, as I couldn't sit and couldn't get my grip. We turned on the jets and it spurred a massive contraction. I leaned over the side and yelled into my (now completely wet) pillow. Ryan saw me sinking in the water and later told me he had about two seconds of inner-panic because he thought I was going to drown. He got in the water with me to help me stay afloat. With his swim trunks, hairy chest, and beard, he looked exactly like the men in the 70's–era photos in the natural birth books! Nice!

It wasn't long before the doc came in and examined me again. She expressed that things 'sounded' like they were going great! She could probably hear me yelling from 10th Avenue. Again, I kind of knew it was time to push, as that is what my body had been telling me and the pressure was SO intense. Sure enough, I was at 10 cm and it was time to get out of the water.

I got on the bed and they draped a warm blanket on me. The doctor and nurse suggested I try getting on hands and knees. I tried that for a few pushes, and let's just say all modesty was completely out the window at that point. Admittedly, and I know this sounds gross, but I remember thinking, 'Oh man, I'm going to sh*t all over these people.'

Amazingly, I didn't much care, and surprisingly, I didn't do it! After a few contractions, we switched to a side-lying position, which seemed to work better for me.

The doctor, nurse, Ryan, and Marin were so encouraging, cheering me on. This was such an important thing to hear, that I was doing well! It really kept me going during this time. Later, I was to learn that I pushed for about 45 minutes. The pain of the contractions was gone, but pushing was certainly physically challenging. The OB used oil and a bit of massage to prevent tearing and showed me where to push— this was very effective. After several rounds of contractions and pushing, the OB told me they could see the baby's head. Ryan was making sounds of awe—he could see the baby emerging!!

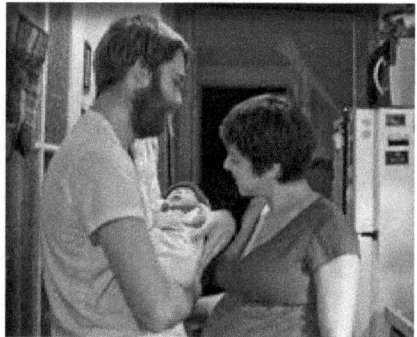

Ryan, Lori, and Emmett. Photo courtesy of Elissa A. Betterbid.

I remember asking if he had hair—yes, he sure did. He was hairy like daddy.

At this integral point, it was Ryan's expressions of amazement that I concentrated on. The sound of his voice made all the difference, and I pushed with renewed vigor. The contractions couldn't come fast enough! Finally, after a couple more contractions and pushes, I heard the baby make a little yelp—yes! He wasn't even all the way out and was already crying!

In the next moment, I felt a release of pressure and Ryan pulled the baby out all the way and cut the cord. Emmett was born at 6:14 a.m., December 3rd—pink and healthy, thank goodness. When he handed the little squirming baby to me, I was in a state of complete astonishment. It was the most amazing moment of my life.

So, all in all, I had pretty much 'textbook' labor, with the active part lasting about 14 hours or so. Emmett was 7 lbs, 15 oz at birth (FYI, at the last of the many ultrasounds I had, three days before his birth, they estimated his weight at 8 lbs 6 oz...go figure). But Emmett grew into a big boy right away; he weighed in at 12 lbs at his four-week pediatrician visit. He's definitely a tit man! Every day we think about how blessed we are to have him. I am now spreading the word on natural childbirth to every couple I know: You CAN do it!!

22

The Surprising Joy of Natural Childbirth

By Lisa Lavoie Gaylord

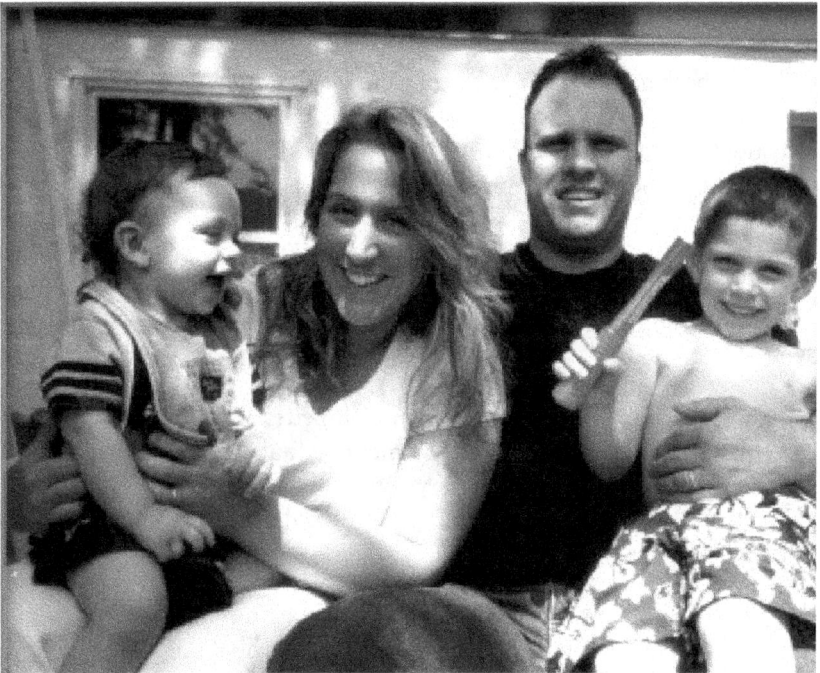

Lisa and Eric with sons Caleb and Eric

I decided to get educated about natural childbirth after the birth of my first child. It was a 20½–hour labor and I had pre-eclampsia, although my OB didn't tell me at the time. It wasn't until I was pregnant with my second son that a new OB at the same clinic informed me it was in my file. Prior to delivery, I spent a full week back and forth to Danbury hospital for induction due to my condition. Each day would be spent alternating between Prepadyl treatments and Pitocin. After a week, we had enough, and I informed the hospital that I would be back when I went into labor on my own.

Labor and delivery were both extremely difficult. I was in so much pain and uninformed of natural pain relieving techniques. Eventually, I requested an epidural. Upon receiving the epidural, my dilation progress came to a complete halt. The baby's heart rate began to drop, as I ran a fever due to meconium. I felt like a pincushion, with all of the different IV's in my arms. I was too exhausted to push, and both the baby and placenta were pulled out with forceps. After the birth, I felt too drugged and weary to enjoy him, and my son spent the next few days in the NICU.

Immediately after this first birth experience, I swore I would never do it that way again. I felt like a total failure. After a couple of years, I decided to start reading up on natural childbirth and doulas. The more I learned, the less anxiety I had about giving birth.

When I became pregnant again, I contacted a doula very early in my pregnancy. We talked about the ideal natural childbirth experience and she reassured me that she would be my ally in the delivery room. Even with the newfound support, I still opted to have my son in the hospital because of the close call with almost losing my older son. While I prepared for my second birth, I read a book called *Maternal Fitness* by Julie Tupler. This book taught me many exercises (besides the kegels), which helped me strengthen the specific abdominal muscles that I needed to help push the baby out.

When it was time for my second labor, I felt better prepared. As soon as my water broke (late at night in bed), we met my doula, Kathy, at the hospital. My contractions were coming very close together. We had immediately requested a birthing room with a labor tub and I was able to labor in the water almost the entire time.

My doula and husband were both very encouraging, but my doula really got me through it. I was able to stay focused throughout, largely due to Kathy's support. She was truly wonderful. She totally respected and supported my wishes, and she stood up to the doctors and nurses when they repeatedly offered drugs. When the pain was getting pretty intense, Kathy kneaded a tennis ball into my lower back and gave me head and hand massages. She also taught my husband the correct technique, so he could join in. She had a hot rice pack that she would put behind my neck while I was laboring in the tub and spoke soothing words about the baby. We kept a soothing, quiet atmosphere in the birthing room, with the lights turned down low and soft music playing. Family would periodically check in, but we kept it to a minimum. During the labor, I was in a peaceful, tranquil state, thanking God for giving me a wonderful experience, which was the total opposite of my first one.

Laboring in the water really helped speed things up; my entire labor and delivery was only three hours and 45 minutes. When it came time to push, the doctor was yelling at me to stop pushing. I felt like I literally could've pushed my baby out in one push, but the doctor felt I would've torn badly. I listened to her and pushed in three pushes, and had minimal tearing. Afterward, the doctor congratulated me on being one of the strongest women she had ever seen push out a baby. I told her I was really strong because of what I learned in *Maternal Fitness*. I was a far cry from the terrified weakling that couldn't even push out the placenta without the help of forceps my first time around.

I love that I was immediately able to breastfeed my son, and we were both alert and happy. When the nurse was pushing Percocet on me after delivery, I smiled and said, "Two Motrin will be fine, thanks." I recovered so much faster with my natural delivery, up and walking around within 15 minutes. I was so proud of myself for doing what I knew was the best thing for me, and most importantly, for my baby. In fact, I believe that delivering my son naturally was possibly my proudest and most joyful moment.

I think every pregnant woman should at least be open to learning about natural childbirth. Reading books and talking to midwives and doulas can help answer questions and ease the anxiety a woman might have. Educating oneself about the risks of medication during labor is helpful as well. Listening to your body when it needs a break is essential to having a good outcome. Rest is absolutely crucial. Staying in shape is important, and I believe a book like *Maternal Fitness*, which shares safe exercises for pregnancy and teaches techniques that will make delivery so much easier, can really help a woman feel prepared for the physical challenges of labor and delivery.

Part IV

Natural Vaginal Birth
After Cesarean

23

VBAC

It is an exciting time for pregnant women in America. It seems like more and more research is coming to light that supports a woman's right to choose the kind of birthing experience she feels most comfortable with, and there is a palpable feeling of change in the air. Women who have had a previous Cesarean section and desire to birth naturally are finally getting more support, and the former "Once a Cesarean, always a Cesarean" era appears to be coming to an end. Even the federal government has taken a side, urging for a decrease in Cesarean sections. In the 2010 Healthy People Report, the U.S. Department of Health and Human Services "set a goal to triple the VBAC rate—acknowledging the cost to pregnant women and healthcare resources of a policy that promotes unnecessary Cesarean sections" (Wagner, 2006, p. 35). This is a positive step, but I still have not seen any bumper stickers stating: *Uncle Sam Wants You to VBAC!*

There is more good news. According to the Center for Disease Control's 2010 report on maternal and infant health statistics …

The cesarean delivery rate declined for the first year in more than a decade to 32.8 percent of all births in 2010, from 32.9 percent in 2009. The percentage of births that were delivered by Cesarean had risen steadily from 1996 through 2009, although the pace of increase had slowed somewhat in recent years (2010).

Clearly, change is in the air!

Still, VBAC is one of the more controversial and polarizing birthing topics today. One mom I know who recently had a successful VBAC told me the pressure from family and friends to agree to a planned section almost won out. Another close friend was pressured to "take advantage of modern medicine and there's a reason these medications were invented." She did her homework, took her birthing preparations seriously, stuck to her convictions, and ended up having the drug-free, satisfying VBAC she wanted. Women desiring to VBAC naturally need to arm themselves with data and plan carefully to protect their rights to the kind of birthing experience they desire.

First and foremost, women need to be aware that there are times when a Cesarean section is necessary and life saving. In emergencies, technology can be key to a positive outcome. C-sections were invented to save lives and certainly have a place in the world of obstetrics. Unfortunately, Cesarean sections and the medical interventions associated with them have become so "normalized" the risks have been seriously downplayed to the detriment of millions of women who have suffered from a host of unexpected, unnecessary side effects, such as excessive pain, bowel obstruction, infertility, miscarriage, negative reactions to the anesthesia, postpartum depression, difficulty bonding with newborn, and even death. As certified childbirth educator and doula Henci Goer puts it in her enlightening book *Obstetric Myths versus Research Realities: A Guide to the Medical Literature* (p. 23), "Cesareans are neither safe nor easy" and should be avoided.

One of the greatest obstacles for women planning to VBAC is fear of uterine rupture. It is crucial for these moms to look to the research. Years ago, most Cesarean incisions were made vertically into the uterus, and because "they were made through the uterine muscle, these incisions occasionally rupture during pregnancy ... the force of labor contractions presumably adds additional stress" (Goer, 1995, p. 41). However, since the 1970s, lower uterine segment transverse incisions became the standard. These lower incisions are in an area that is mostly connective tissue. "Study after study has shown, it rarely gives way, and when it does, the separation is usually like opening a zipper; neat, bloodless, and benign" (Goer, 1995, p. 41). The

"Put your energy into thinking about what you WANT, instead of what you DON'T want. Erase negative thoughts! Ask yourself, what message have I learned about birth? Have I heard over and over again that birth is impossible or too hard? Do I have only crazy Hollywood versions of birth instilled in me? Did I hear repeatedly as I grew up, from my mother and other women, that birth was "horrible," "too hard," or "almost killed" them? These messages are deeply rooted and potentially dangerous to normal birth. They can block the birth passageway. Given the opportunity to explore those messages, women can rewind the negative tape and fill it with positive messages and affirmations...but first they have to understand what their existing tape is. This is especially true for women planning VBAC, who may have an entire difficult birth experience on their tape."—Catherine Gallagher, CNM

Connecticut Childbirth & Women's Center

National Institutes of Health reported in a 2004 study that "uterine ruptures occur in fewer than one percent of those who attempted VBAC" (Landon, 2004, p. 2655). Still, uterine rupture is a valid concern and one has to weigh the benefits with the risks before she commits to a VBAC.

To ensure a successful VBAC, a mom needs to prepare herself. First step is finding a confident care provider with ample experience. In her book *The Thinking Woman's Guide to a Better Birth*, Henci Goer explains … "almost all complications occur in women who have repeat Cesareans, so the better your odds of vaginal birth, the lower your chances of experiencing them. You want an encouraging caregiver who performs only medically indicated repeat Cesareans and who has a VBAC rate of 70 percent or more" (1999, p. 171).

Furthermore, studies have shown an increased risk of uterine rupture and repeat Cesarean when labor was induced or augmented by synthetic oxytocin, otherwise known as Pitocin. Epidurals also put laboring women at a greater risk for emergency C-sections. Epidurals are known to:

… cause episodes of abnormally slow fetal heart rate in about 10 percent of laboring women. The most reliable sign that a scar has opened and is causing the baby problems is abnormally slow fetal heart rate, which means that an epidural puts you at greater risk of an emergency Cesarean for suspected scar separation (Goer, 1999, 172).

For many years, women were lead to believe that once they had a Cesarean they would have no other choice for subsequent births but a repeat Cesarean. In 2004 the New England Journal of Medicine published a study of 18,000 women showing "75 percent of VBACs are successful (no surgical intervention needed)" (Greene, 2004). Luckily, significant research has overridden this myth, and women are now being offered a choice in most areas of the United States.

24

The Strength of My Scar: The Incredible VBAC of James

By Lisl Dunlop

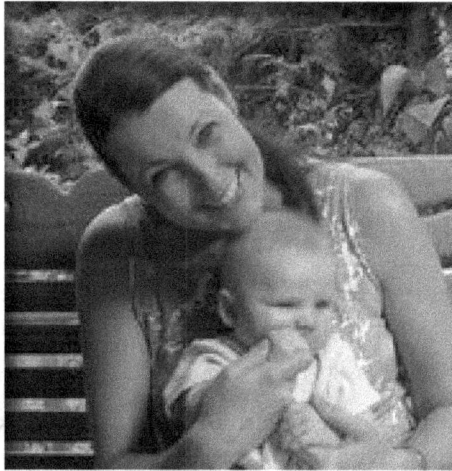

Lisl and James

It has been over two years since Jamie's birth in March 2009, but my memories of that time are still incredibly vivid. It was one of the most amazing, momentous, uplifting events of my life, made all the more precious by what had gone before.

Four years earlier, my daughter, Audrey, was born six weeks premature by emergency Cesarean section in a New York City hospital. The end of that pregnancy was marked by complications, and I was comfortable that the surgery was medically necessary. Yet, when I finally became pregnant with James, I wanted to do things differently. I wanted to experience the wonder of childbirth personally and actively, and to have the joy and victory of seeing and holding my baby as he was born.

After starting out my prenatal care in a traditional OB practice, I became more and more uneasy as the months went by. Although initially expressing support for a vaginal birth after Cesarean (VBAC) and natural childbirth in principle, my doctors did little to investigate my prior history, discuss the risks and benefits of birth alternatives, or discuss hospital protocols and what to expect. In a series of rushed appointments (following extended and unexplained periods in the waiting room), I tried to ask questions. The answers, when they came, were not encouraging. Although I could try to labor without drugs, they told me, in their experience the vast majority of their patients need epidural pain relief, and they didn't see how I would be different. They suggested that another Cesarean would be much easier on me and asked me to schedule a section for a few days after my due date "to get it on the calendar." The last straw came when I received a call from the practice to tell me I had been scheduled for a section a week prior to my due date without my knowledge or agreement.

Even before this, I had started to investigate alternatives, talking with midwives, doctors, doulas, and other women who had successfully had VBACs. A Hypnobirthing class I took in January 2009 led me to the local chapter of the International Cesarean Awareness Network (ICAN) and the wealth of resources and support there. I learned that finding supportive people and a supportive place in which to give birth is the most important part of ensuring a positive birth experience, and many of the most positive stories I heard ended at Danbury.

I made an appointment to meet the midwives at the Connecticut Childbirth and Women's Center, with only six weeks to go in my pregnancy. Upon meeting with Cathy Gallagher, I immediately felt that here was someone who understood all my hopes and fears. Cathy showed me some letters she had received from other mothers who attempted VBACs with her. The one that most affected me was one from a mother who ended up with a C-section, but nevertheless expressed gratitude for being given the opportunity to labor and try to give birth naturally. Our meeting left me convinced that this group understood and supported the emotion involved in birth, as well as the mechanics. As I was leaving, I tentatively asked another question about the risk of uterine rupture. After reiterating the basic statistics, Cathy surprised me by telling me not to ignore the mind-body connection, and instead of worrying about rupture, to focus on the strength of my uterine scar. I knew I was in the right place. Despite the hour's drive from my home, I transferred my care, with only a month to go before Jamie's "due date."

My official "due date" was March 9. As that day came and went, I agonized over the upcoming discussion at my next appointment about scheduling a repeat C-section at 41 weeks (as required by the back-up obstetricians and the hospital). To my great relief, I never made it to that appointment. As I lay in bed early in the morning of March 11, I woke up with some cramping. After this happened two or three times, my waters broke. It was about 6:00 a.m. After I cleaned myself up, I lay back down and tried to rest, but I was too excited at the prospect of the baby finally coming. I went into a frenzy of activity, answering emails, setting my out-of-office messages, finishing final packing for the hospital, and letting family and friends know that it had started. I called my mother in Australia—with the time difference, it was late in the evening—and she was thrilled to hear it was happening at last.

I labored at home all through Wednesday, with a trip up to Danbury for a non-stress test around the middle of the day, which went fine. The surges were coming about every 15 or 20 minutes, with good breaks in between. I practiced Hypnobirthing surge breathing when I needed to and stayed active all day, walking around the house, leaning on the kitchen counters for contractions, sitting on the rocking chair in the baby's room and on the birthing ball in my bedroom, and doing laundry (the bed sheets from my waters' breaking!) and other menial tasks in between. Although I wasn't hungry, I tried to eat small meals to keep up my strength. It became hard to focus on anything for any length of time, but time seemed to pass quite quickly.

Labor continued all through Wednesday night, with the surges becoming more intense, but still very spaced apart. I took a relaxing bath with candles, and then tried to rest in bed, but found it harder to cope with the surges lying down on my left side, so I went into the baby's room to sit on the rocking chair and let my husband, Giff, get some rest. By this time, it was daytime in Australia again, so I called my mother. She once again told me the stories of my birth and my brother's birth, both of which had been very long. Despite this, she had found the sensations of birth completely manageable and ultimately had successful vaginal deliveries. We joked about how a doctor in New Zealand 40 years ago had told her she had a "slow womb." Finally, I called my doula, Margaret, around 2:00 a.m. to come and keep me company, and she sat near me talking when I wanted to and monitoring how far apart the surges were coming. Although they were getting quite strong, the surges were completely manageable with a combination of relaxation, surge breathing, and position changes. By 4:00 a.m., I was starting to get concerned about how I would handle an hour in the car and was thinking of heading to the hospital, but the surges were still around 10 minutes apart. Sarah Najamy, who had been at the hospital all night in case I came in, discouraged me from coming in too early. Since I only had a few hours to wait before I had been asked to come in anyway (8:00 a.m.), we stayed at home.

At about 7:00 a.m., we loaded up the car and headed up to Danbury. At this point, my waters had been broken for more than 24 hours and I was preparing myself to be told that I needed to have a C-section when I arrived. I listened to "Rainbow Relaxation" in the car to help calm myself and manage the intense surges I was having. Because they were still fairly spaced out, I only had about five contractions on the 50-minute car trip and was able to walk up to the L&D ward on the second floor of the hospital.

When I arrived around 8:00 a.m., they showed me straight into a labor room, where I met with Cathy Gallagher and Sarah Najami. I sat on the bed, so they could monitor the baby's heart rate for 20 minutes or so. Cathy Gallagher examined me—my cervix had dilated by about 4 centimeters. This was a little discouraging—all that time and effort for only 4 centimeters! I had blood taken, so my white count could be checked (for infection), and I continued to labor sitting on the bed for another 30 minutes, waiting for Cathy to return with the back-up OB, Dr. Whitcombe. To my enormous relief, Dr. W. said the baby was doing fine, she had reviewed my records and I was a perfect VBAC candidate, and there was no reason why I should not continue. There was no mention of a C-section. I felt like I had been let out of jail!

I continued to labor throughout the day on Thursday. I hoped that once I was at the hospital things would move more quickly, but it was a long, slow process. We created a peaceful, soothing atmosphere, with our iPod and speakers playing relaxation albums and classical music. The blinds were drawn and lights were low, and for much of the time, the only people in the room were me, Giff, and Margaret. Cathy G appeared at various points throughout the day, gently suggesting position changes and things to relieve the pressure (wet towels heated in the microwave and placed around my stomach and back and underneath me were bliss!) Throughout the day, I tried a variety of different positions for labor—in the shower, the tub, on the ball or rocking chair, on the bed.

We had a wonderful L&D nurse, Lois, looking after us that day. Towards the end of my pregnancy, I had given a lot of thought to my birth preferences and written a birth plan. Margaret made sure that Lois had the plan, and it was clear she had read it and was happy to support my choices. She seemed to understand quickly that we were very prepared for this birth and did not try to interpose herself into my circle of comfort or to suggest checks or interventions. Yet, her positive attitude and support were very important. At one point I remember laboring in the tub and joking that I would need an epidural if things got too much more intense. Lois overheard from where she was charting over near the bed and commented, "Oh, you won't need an epidural." To hear someone other than my cheerleaders say that gave me tremendous confidence that I was coping well and could do it.

At about 2:30 p.m., I got restless with our peaceful atmosphere, so I got dressed and went for a walk around the post-partum unit with Giff, occasionally leaning on the wall as I had contractions. We stopped to look into the nursery "for inspiration"—as usual, only one or two babies were there; Danbury really encourages rooming in and most babies were with their families. On the way back to the room, we stopped in the hallway to call my four-year-old daughter, Audrey. She asked why baby brother was taking so long to come out and suggested we tickle him to get him to move, which cracked us both up.

When we returned to the room, my labor picked up. I sat on the birthing ball and leaned over pillows on the bed, rotating my hips to cope with the intense contractions. At this point, I had a contraction, or multiple contractions one after another, lasting for about three minutes. I was so surprised at this, saying, "It won't end" over and over, as I tried to do surge breathing and kept running out of air. Then it occurred to me that maybe things were moving and the baby might be coming at last. I was suddenly overwhelmed with emotion. At that moment, Anne-Marie, the student midwife, came in to check on me—she took one look at my face and panicked, thinking I was in terrible pain. I tried to tell here that it wasn't pain, but I think it gave her a shock. While leaning forward to deal with that contraction, the monitor had slipped down and was not monitoring the baby's heart rate, although the contractions registered. Once they adjusted the heart-rate monitor and checked the baby through a few more contractions, everyone calmed down.

Unfortunately, it was not quite the end, although things did get much more intense from then on. Cathy checked me (this was only the second cervical check) and found that I was dilating unevenly. She suggested that I labor on my side to encourage the head to push down on the cervix. This was the worst part of the labor, with very painful contractions, and I vomited in the middle of them. Giff and Margaret encouraged and held me through it all.

So much time had passed since we arrived that a new back-up OB had come on shift. She chose this time to introduce herself—I was so focused on what I was doing, it was all I could do to acknowledge her. Cathy suggested that I submit to another cervical check—the subtext was that I needed to get the new OB comfortable with the situation. To be fair, I had been in labor for about 36 hours by this point, nearly 10 in the hospital, and had that "prior C-section " cloud hanging over my head. So, I submitted to the cervical check and was happy to hear that I was close to complete "with a lip." A little more creative laboring (including Cathy manually pushing back the lip while I was on the birthing chair) and I was ready for the next stage.

Nothing I'd read or heard prepared me for the intensity of the pushing stage. I'm sure everyone experiences it differently, but for me, those moments were like nothing I'd ever anticipated. Earlier in the labor, while I was in the tub, Cathy had commented that I was handling things very well and seemed very controlled, but that I had to be prepared for the experience to get "bigger than I was" at some point and that I needed to let go. This scared me a bit, but it still didn't prepare me for what it was like. The sensations were so intense that I could not even open my eyes. A mirror had been placed at the end of the bed for me to watch my baby emerging, but after only a quick glance, I shut my eyes again—sensory overload! The pushing contractions were so intense that I started to scream with them. Then I heard Cathy's voice telling me to keep my voice low and bring the baby down with short grunts. I hung onto her voice through two or three more surges, as my body stretched and widened around my baby, and he moved down little bit by little bit. It was not painful, so much as surprising. I felt like the universe was being turned inside out and thought

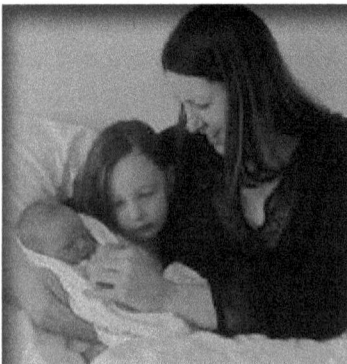
Lisl, Audrey, and James

I could see stars. I kept muttering, "This is surreal, this is surreal" between my contractions, unable to process all the sensations.

Through it all I was aware of gentle hands holding my legs and pouring oil on my perineum, and supporting me there. At one point I felt some burning at the front of my vagina, and then the sensation stopped as someone pressed James' head back towards my perineum. With my eyes still tight shut,

I reached down and felt his head emerging. Along with the midwives, I cradled his head as it emerged from my body, and in the next surge, his body followed. Eager hands helped mine bring him up to my chest and covered us with warm blankets. "Precious, so precious" I repeated, over and over. People were laughing and crying. Giff leaned over and kissed me, Margaret was beaming. I held onto James for dear life—nothing would make me let go of him.

25

Never As Planned, But As It Should Be

By Jennifer McCann

I hope the details can come to me, as time has passed, and I am busy these days with Colin (5), Corey (3) and Sarah (1). We all come to our experiences, especially our births, with preconceived notions, customs, and expectations. My first child was born in October 2005. I came into that pregnancy as: a daughter of a mother who birthed all three of us naturally in the 1970's, a registered nurse for eight years, five of which were working in obstetrics, four years as a childbirth educator, and a student working on my Masters to become a certified nurse midwife. I ended up changing to get my Masters in nursing education instead. However, during my school clinical practicums, I worked at Connecticut Childbirth and Women's Center as a midwifery student. Little did I know, I would end up birthing my second and third children with them.

I felt like I was part of an experiment during my first pregnancy, labor, and even post-partum experience. I had read so many books to aid in my teaching of childbirth classes and knew about using as many resources as possible. I had already been going to a midwife in White Plains, New York, several years before getting pregnant. It is funny to be a nurse in the profession, and then to be going through it all yourself. Some days I felt like I knew nothing. Other days I felt like I knew too much.

I think people found it funny that I chose to take a childbirth class for my first birth. I wanted to experience it all, plus I feel the classes are and should be geared more for the partners. I actually learned a lot of resources available for pain and diet in pregnancy. I got a meditation CD from the teacher, about 20 minutes long, which I did on my lunch break or at home each day. It focused on full body relaxation and sort of walked you calmly through labor and birth. I took prenatal yoga classes a couple days a week with both of my first two pregnancies. They helped with strength, body awareness, and relaxation. I also asked my husband, Dan, to read *The Birth Partner* by Penny Simkin, which he dutifully did. It was very sweet, seeing it on his bed stand. I chose not to have a doula with my first pregnancy, but when the time came, I wished I had at least someone in addition to Dan who could labor "with me." One wonderful book I found was *Mind Over Labor* by Carl Jones—it's old and hard to find, but it was so helpful. It has all these meditations for labor. Another great resource was *Spiritual Midwifery* by Ina May Gaskin. It is filled with positive, wonderful experiences of childbirth. I had to look over the hippy nature of some parts of the book. Contractions are described as "rushes" and labors are described as enjoyable experiences by the women telling their stories, not as fear and pain and suffering. I also found William Sears' *Birth Book* to be very informative and to have lots of tips, ideas, and options for dealing with the pain in labor.

I compiled a list of ideas and strategies for labor—like my own toolbox of what to do in labor. I knew I might need Dan to say, "There are things we haven't tried yet," in case the labor was long or I felt helpless, he could pull out the list. Included in that list of ideas were: relaxing songs on a CD, tennis balls to massage my back, lavender scented lotion, and a rice sock—a sock filled with rice and tied closed, which can be microwaved and used as moist heat.

One thing, which might sound crazy, was that I made a deal with my husband and the midwives that even if I ask for drugs or an epidural, not to let me have it. I have witnessed so many women who were so dedicated to giving birth naturally, and then when the medication was so readily available, they would get an epidural. I knew that every woman has a moment of "I just can't do it anymore." One lactation consultant I worked with told me that every woman has a moment of weakness and even she, who chose to give birth at home, was asking her midwife for an epidural. I just knew that for myself I had to not think of it as an option. I also knew deep down that the midwife would do what was best with me at that time. I trusted the midwives completely.

My labor started on a Saturday night, my actual due date, October 22nd. I felt very mild abdominal tightening all night, irregular. I stayed in bed, did not wake my husband, and listened to my iPod with a relaxing playlist I had made ahead of time. Sunday morning we went and got bagels, while I tried to ignore the contractions. We went for a long walk that day through the park across the street—one of my fondest memories of the labor. It was a crisp autumn day, my husband held my hand, we stopped and swayed during the contractions with my head on his shoulder. We laughed and talked about names, and if it would be a boy or girl, and how our life was going to change. The beautiful thing is that between contractions you really are totally pain free, so I tried to focus on and remember that time, especially in early labor.

During labor I had a few "mantras" that I said to myself. One that really helped was, "I can do anything for a minute." Also, I told myself, "It's just one day in your life, Jen." Another thing that carried me through a lot of that first birth was a brief news story I had seen in September 2005, just after the tsunami hit Indonesia. This amazing woman gave birth, while stuck, by herself, in the top of a tree! That's all I knew about the story, no more details, no photo, but that woman carried me through the birth, along with the thought of the millions of women now and in the past who have done this. I convinced myself that women are designed to birth babies. That's it; it's as simple as that!

Sunday afternoon we watched a funny movie (*Old School*) together, while I rocked on the birth ball and my husband rubbed my lower back. I actually hardly watched the movie, but just watched the counter timer on the DVD player. The contractions were steadily two minutes apart. I called the midwife and she took a while to call me back (she was with another birth), so I started to panic. Looking back, I think this waiting accelerated my pain. I went to the hospital around 6:00 p.m. and wouldn't you know? My contractions totally stopped when I got there. I should have stayed home!

I was checked by the midwife Sunday evening and was only 1 or 2 cm. It was hard because I sensed that they must get stronger, but they were already every two minutes for hours and hours. I chose to go home. The contractions were milder and more spaced out all night, and my husband and I were so tired by then, we just each passed out on a couch in our living room. I was lying in one position for hours, afraid to move. By Monday morning, the contractions started up again, and I went in to the midwife's office at 10:00 a.m. for my pre-scheduled appointment. Again, I was about 1 or 2 cm! So I went home again, exhausted, with instructions to take some Benadryl, so that I could try to get some rest.

I went home and showered, thank God for showering. I would not say I had "back labor" because the pain was in front, but I could not tolerate being on my back. Monday afternoon, I got into this rhythm of rocking back and forth on my knees for a couple hours, and then resting in child's pose between contractions. While the Benadryl was in my system, it was a pretty horrible feeling. I'd wake in pain, but feel so groggy between contractions. The contractions were definitely stronger by then and coming every two minutes again.

Around this time I had this overwhelming feeling of needing women around me, women who were strong, and women who had given birth before. I really didn't have anyone to call. My sister and mom live far away, and my friends and family nearby were either working or home with their own babies. Throughout all of this, my husband was so unbelievably awesome! He never left my side. He massaged my lower back, supported me emotionally and physically, fed me food and drinks, gave me words of encouragement, and often was just silently present. He utilized all the techniques we had talked about during the pregnancy. This experience totally brought us closer. But he was getting tired, too. I joked after the birth that he looked worse than me! After three days of labor, he had a beard, had not eaten, and was exhausted. Looking back, a doula or other labor support would have given him a break and given us both the support we needed.

Monday evening I called the midwife to update her on my progress. We had been in touch every few hours. She had me come in … again. Each car ride was tough. I sat in the front seat facing the back of the car, on my knees, holding onto the headrest and had a pillow under my belly. I brought a towel and bucket in case of vomiting.

Once in the hospital, I had the support of more people that I had craved at home. My "favorite" midwife from the group, Robyn, was there. And, coincidentally, another midwife from the practice was working per diem that night as an RN in labor and delivery, so she was my nurse. That was lucky! Upon admission I was about 5 centimeters dilated. With all three of my labors, I feel like I had all the right people around me, like the stars were in line.

In the hospital they allowed me to move around. I continued to use visualization, riding the contractions like waves or pretending I was floating in the ocean; using different positions: standing, leaning forward on the birth ball, swaying with my husband, rocking on all fours in the shower tub. I tried the Jacuzzi one time, but did not like it at all; in fact, I jumped right out. I felt out of my rhythm that I had been in at home, and I did not like the feeling of my belly floating in the water. A little later, I tried it again, and it was better, much more relaxing. I also showered again in the hospital. Showers were so great: the rhythm of the water beating on me and the relaxation of the warm water really helped.

The trusting relationship between the midwife and me was formed in office visits throughout the pregnancy. When the midwife asked me to do lunges and nipple stimulation to move the labor along, I did it. I lunged, squatted, rocked, got on all fours, stopped pushing, pushed. Whatever they said, I did it. I had such unbelievable faith in them to do what was best for me. I trusted their expertise and surrendered to the labor.

Finally, late in the night, I was about 9.5 cm dilated. Apparently I tend to get stuck at 9.5 cm, it's called an "anterior lip" of the cervix, and it happened with all three of my labors. The midwife tried everything to help the cervix open to 10 cm, and even used some low dose Pitocin. After about 52 hours of labor, I ended up having a C-section! I was getting a little paranoid at the end there because the midwife was going in and out of the room. I knew she was considering a C-section. The baby's head was not descending. Our baby was posterior (face up) and starting to show some distress, while I pushed on and off, and I was still at 9.5 cm for hours and hours. I was sad, but I was also exhausted. The obstetrician was called in, and she said very simply, "I heard you have been doing such a wonderful job." She was the one doing the surgery, and this was the first time we met, but she was very comforting with those simple words. I warned the midwife, "Hey, I may have postpartum depression because of this." I was half joking, but knew that I really, really did not want to have a C-section! I got an epidural, which was not painful at all compared to labor, and was brought into the operating room. I felt slightly like it was an out of body experience. I was, of course, numb, and I just felt like it was not me they were doing the surgery on. I asked the midwife to tell me exactly what they were doing through the surgery, as if I was a patient and not myself. I had assisted in many C-sections before.

When I heard that first cry and, "It's a boy!" it was such a relief! My husband held him and I got to touch and see him, but not hold him yet. He was gorgeous—big full lips and blond hair. Colin Patrick was 8 lbs 14 oz.

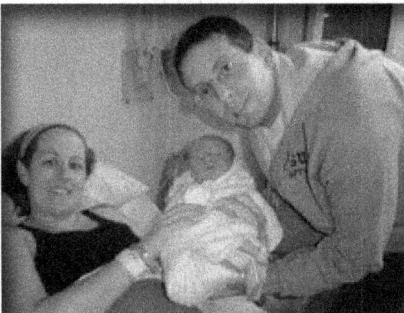
Jennifer and Dan with Colin Patrick

The immediate love was overwhelming. After the surgery, I was wheeled into the recovery room, as they brought him to the nursery because his breathing was slightly distressed. This was a horrible feeling, and I grabbed my nurse by the scrubs and was like, "Bring me my baby." (I'm exaggerating). At this point I knew what can happen— he goes to the nursery, looks fine, but then hangs out under the warmer and gets a bath, and then it is change of shift, etc. etc. I had an overwhelming feeling about carrying him for nine months, and then just wanting to hold him forever—this feeling lasted months after he was born! Anyway, the midwife came to see me in the recovery room and went to the nursery herself to get him for me. It was about an hour that I did not see him.

Of course, I was so upset about having the C-section. However, I realized that Dan and I, and the midwife, had given it every possible chance. I knew that I did all that I could do on my end, and although it was a long, hard labor, it was all worth it. We even talked about it at my two-week visit, and she allowed me to cry and grieve and mourn the loss of a vaginal delivery. It helped that she told me that she allowed the labor to go on longer than she would have liked because she knew how important it was for me to not have a C-section. The midwife allowed for this time at our two-week visit to talk and review the birth details. She realized the importance of it.

It was very hard that the labor did not go as planned—except it really never does. And I found it very difficult that people would say, "as long as the baby is healthy." It just sounds so condescending to me. Of course, that is a mother's most important goal! Having a satisfying birth experience is definitely second on the list. For me, the process of labor and the birth were almost as important as the outcome. One cool thing was that I had this feeling of being the most powerful, strongest woman after enduring that labor—everything else seemed so easy compared to that.

When Colin was two, I was pregnant again and determined to have a VBAC (vaginal birth after Cesarean). I was told by midwives and doctors that I had to be okay with the possibility of having the same long labor that could end in a C-section. For me, it was worth the try, and I was willing to go through it all again. It was necessary for me to really try again.

My original midwife group no longer took my insurance, so I decided to see a doctor from work who I knew did a lot of successful VBACs. I knew I needed someone committed to trying a VBAC. It was also important for me to give birth in the appropriate hospital environment with back up to provide a C-section quickly if the need arises. By about 30 weeks, I could not go to the doctor any more—I tried, I really did, but I just missed the midwives so much. The doctor was a bit of a hike to New York City, and most visits I would wait and wait in the office—sometimes for two hours to have a 10–minute visit. He promoted gaining less weight to "make a smaller baby," but never gave me practical advice or reviewed what I was doing already, as far as exercise and diet. By the way, I gained 40 pounds with Colin, 25 pounds with the second baby, and 20 pounds with the third. I got comments such as, "I'm disappointed in your weight gain this week," and his partner even said to me, " I didn't know you were a hippy!" when I told him I wanted a natural birth. I worked with both these obstetricians at the hospital, and they were fine providers, but they seemed to miss the point, and I feel they were not comfortable with natural childbirth. They also did not have the time to spend in the office, probably due to insurance, etc. Soooooo, after much deliberation I ended up with the midwives in Danbury—it was a little far, but they took my insurance, and I was moving slightly closer to them a month before my due date anyway. What a sense of peace I felt after the first visit! They spent time chatting, listening, and welcoming me in.

This time I had a friend named Marci agree to be a doula for me. I had met Marci through my son's playgroup, and she was passionate about natural childbirth. Apparently, she had always wanted to be a doula, but had not had any formal training for it, but the timing and the price (free) was right. My husband and I met with her while I was pregnant and talked about how our last labor went and our wishes for this time around. She has a calm vibe about her.

I woke up on Wednesday morning around 7:00 a.m., three days before my due date, and was feeling abdominal tightening every five to ten minutes. I went for a walk in my neighborhood, while my husband was still home and listened to some of my favorite songs on my IPod. The contractions were getting stronger, and as I got closer to home, I had to stop and breathe through them.

I called my step-mom, Lynn (aka Grandma), to come over early on to watch Colin, but I sent my husband to work, figuring it might take a long time. I went upstairs to my bedroom, while Grandma played with Colin downstairs. I sat on a large birth (exercise) ball, with my upper body resting on the bed and watched TV. I breathed through the contractions, nice, slow, even breaths in and out, with a big breath before and after the contractions, while rocking side to side. I tried to rest and distract myself with *Regis and Kelly*, then *Rachel Ray*, but by the time *The View* was on, I did not want to be alone anymore. During that time, I spoke with Dan at work, and I also talked to my sister Liz in Minnesota. She was at work and dying to come be with me. She ended up calling me back and said she was getting on a plane after work!

By 11:00 a.m., I called Dan to come home and Marci to come over. I went downstairs and walked around, stopping with every contraction and leaning over on the back of the couch and the kitchen counter, staying calm around Grandma and Colin. For me, my contractions were two minutes apart all along, so with each labor, it was always hard to tell when to go in. Dan came home and Marci came over about 12:30 p.m. I did not want to go in for fear of being sent home. The midwife helped guide me over the phone. We drove the 35–minute ride to the office together in the car. Marci was in the back seat with me. I rode the whole way backwards on my knees. They examined me in the office and I was already 5cm. The plan was to deliver in the hospital because I was a VBAC.

The midwives let me walk around the birth center upstairs from their office, no one was laboring there, and let my labor progress a while before admitting me to the hospital. I continued to walk, but felt like I was getting tired. Marci and my husband basically just were very present and quietly supporting me, rubbing my lower back, reminding me to take sips of juice and eat a little. I remember Marci kept suggesting I sit on the toilet, and I felt myself getting irritable, I was probably in transition! For some reason, it felt very uncomfortable for me to sit on the toilet during that time and it was hard to urinate.

The midwives were changing shift at about 5:00 p.m., so they both came up to check on me. While they were there, I had a gush of fluid and blood. Thinking my water broke, we drove over to the office—all four of us got in the car and drove across the street. It was all very calm, though. For me, I did not like it when people were buzzing about around me, talking or getting nervous. I needed that calm energy throughout. I walked up to the unit with the midwife, and they got me settled in a room right away. They checked me and I was 7 centimeters!

Again, I had the anterior lip problem and could not push until I was fully dilated. Also, the baby was posterior, like Colin. The labor nurse and a student nurse, who was working with her, were both great, very laid-back, and they allowed me to "refuse" to be monitored for a bit while I moved around the room. I walked around the room and was muttering to myself, "This is ridiculous" and "Why do women have to do this?" and "I can do this. Women all around the world do this every day, in every country." Once again I had my favorite midwife on call, Cathy, and she was fantastic with trying different positions for laboring and pushing. I was on all fours, squatting, on the toilet, in the bed using the squatting bar, and sitting on a birth stool. I pushed off and on about two hours. Pushing was ridiculously hard! I feel like I made the best progress with the pushes where Dan and I lock arms across the bed, while I stood on the floor squatting and pushing down.

I had a hard time believing I was giving birth vaginally until they told me they could see the head. The midwife explained that after a VBAC a lot of women need to get past the point where they were "stuck" last time. It was so true. Finally, the head was coming out, and I was screaming a loud, high pitched, uncontrollable scream. Cathy locked eyes with me and basically told me to get it together and to slowly let the head come out. What a relief! They put her on my belly and I announced, "It's a girl," as she peed on me. I was shouting over and over, "I did it! I did it!" I put her right to the breast to feed. Amazing! She was born at 9:43 p.m. Coralee Elizabeth weighed just 7 lbs 4 oz, but she came out posterior, so that made for a tough recovery. What an unbelievable experience—I was able to hold and nurse her immediately, something I had missed out on with Colin. She was gorgeous. She was bathed right in the labor room and never left my side during the whole hospital stay.

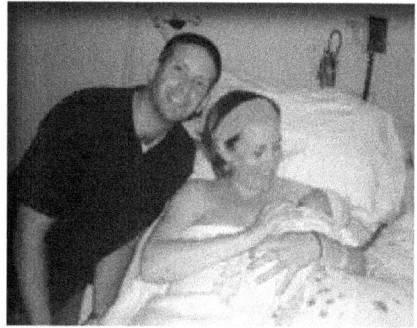

My sister arrived at the airport in New York just as I was giving birth and arrived at the hospital at about 12 midnight Wednesday night. She was so supportive and helpful, and I was so relieved to see her. She ended up staying the whole weekend through Sunday.

The recovery was so much better this time around. My bottom was sore for about two weeks, and ini-

Jennifer and Dan with Coralee Elizabeth

tially I wasn't sure which was better—vaginal birth or C-section. But after two weeks, there was no comparison. This time was so much better, physically and emotionally. The birth was difficult, but again, it felt like everything was in line with how it was supposed to be and I was so proud of myself. When I went back to work after having Coralee, I had a revelation: everything happens for a reason. I had a newfound empathy for my patients who experience either vaginal birth or Cesarean. Maybe that experience was to strengthen my compassion as a nurse.

My third birth was two years later, and, honestly, I felt like I did nothing to prepare, besides walking and trying to keep my weight down. It was hard with two little ones at home. One thing I did do was go to a chiropractor from about 26 weeks on for lower back pain, and she specialized in pregnancy and postpartum care. She did some massage maneuvers, which are supposed to help, so the baby is not posterior. The last couple of weeks I pulled out my *Mind Over Labor* book, and I found some meditations on iTunes. I also sat down and compiled a new toolbox of ideas for dealing with labor.

Again, it felt like the stars were in line for me for the birth. I was due August 16th. My sister and mom came in from Minnesota and Massachusetts the weekend after my due date. Again, last minute, my sister said, "I can't take it, I'm coming for the weekend, and I'll be with you whether you have the baby or not." I swear the baby was waiting for them, and also for the midwife, Cathy, to be on call that weekend.

I felt such pressure to give birth while they were there. We went out for Mexican food for dinner. I also heard you should eat pineapple, have sex, and try castor oil. I tried it all. Well, a half dose of castor oil. My sister and I went for long walks, to walk the baby out. While we walked, we talked about all the things that helped me in my previous two labors—I told her it helps to tell me, "It's just one day of your life," "You can do anything for a minute," and "You are not going to die—you're just having a baby."

Labor started this time about 3:00 a.m. on Sunday morning. I woke up and was having tightening in my abdomen about eight minutes apart. I just laid on my side and watched TV in bed. By about 5:00 a.m., they were getting longer, stronger, and closer together, and I woke up my husband. My mom and sister were sleeping downstairs in the guest room, and I did not want to wake them too early or unnecessarily, so we stayed upstairs. I sat on the birth ball while the rest of the house was still sleeping. My husband got his bag ready.

By 6:30 a.m., we went downstairs to wake my mom and sister. They were both very excited and got busy getting ready for the day. I labored on the birth ball in the living room and again watched a funny movie—this time I half watched *Knocked Up!* I ate an English Muffin with butter. Colin and Corey woke up at 7:30 a.m. My husband went upstairs and got them dressed and ready to go to my cousin's house. It was perfect timing, she arrived as they came downstairs, and they all headed right out the door. The contractions were getting more intense at that time, and I remember trying to pretend, Mommy is fine. As they came down the stairs, I headed up, giving them kisses, and crawling up the stairs as another contraction came.

I headed to the shower with my sister. She was so helpful, timing the contractions, and guiding me through them, telling me when the peak was done, and when they were almost over. That really helped, not to say when it is getting worse, but to only point out that a contraction is easing off.

Something changed in the shower—I guess I was probably in transition, and my sister insisted we go in—I did not want to go for fear of being sent home. I did not feel ready to go in. I was in the shower, on all fours, and I was moaning a lot through the contractions, but my sister says I was grunting and pushing through them. They were also peaking, but then peaking again and getting longer, signs of transition. The other sign of transition I had, in retrospect, was getting emotional and panicking. It was so cool because Liz had listened to all I had said on our walk and really put it into action. I got into a groove with her, and I asked her come in the car with us—my mom followed. Rhythms and rituals are very important in labor—the Penny Simkin book talks a lot about this. I had gotten into a rhythm with the way she was talking me through the contractions. I rode in again in the back seat, on my knees facing the back of the car. The midwife, Cathy, was on call and she planned to meet us at the hospital.

I opted for the hospital this time. The midwives said I could have given birth at the birth center, but I made that choice because I felt I was still a VBAC and a higher risk for a C-section. Plus, I had had such a great experience at the hospital the last time. It just felt like the right place for me. Once at the hospital, Dan and I walked down this hallway, which seemed like the longest hallway ever. I remember stopping at each windowsill to lean over and breathe through the contractions. We got to the hospital room at 9:00 a.m., and Cathy checked me. I was fully dilated, besides the anterior lip again. That was really cool and a total shock me! I thought I still had hours to go. My sister especially was so emotional because it became clear that she would be there for the birth. She would have to leave for the airport by 2:00 p.m. And my mom and husband were there, so it was so perfect!

This time they monitored me briefly, but then let me walk around the room. I sat on the toilet a lot, but mostly just paced in the room. Cathy went to assist in a birth next door and had the nurse not let me push. It felt, at the time, like torture. I just wanted to push! I really was not aware what was going on around me. I was just pacing and leaning over the labor bed, which was raised up higher. The nurse was excellent again this time.

Finally, Cathy came back and that little bit of cervix was gone, so I started to push. I made the most progress pushing lying flat on my back this time. Sarah Katherine was born at 11:00 a.m., after pushing about 20 minutes. She weighed exactly what Colin did: 8 lbs 14 oz. Again I was screaming when she came out that, "I did it" and "It's a girl!" It was so, so, so unbelievable to have my husband, mom, sister, and favorite midwife there with me—and I had a great L&D nurse, too. She, too, was bathed right in the room with me and never left my side until discharge. I had the best hospital stay—no visitors, except Colin and Corey, so I just rested and bonded with beautiful Sarah.

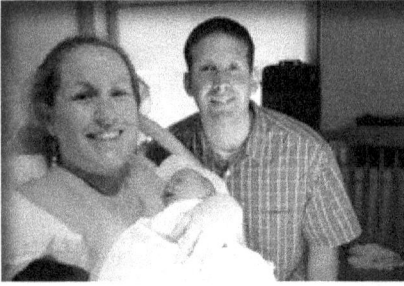

Jennifer and Dan with Sarah Katherine

I loved my labors. I think about them as my passage to motherhood. I really tried to block out any negative birth stories when I was pregnant. Every labor can be told as a horror story. I feel like we as women need to hear more birth stories told in a positive light and support each other with realistic expectations and helpful tips. Those relatively few days of labor I had with all three are nothing compared to the years of "labor" I've had thus far as a mother to three adorable, challenging, wonderful children. I would not change a thing! Nothing went as planned, but everything went as it should be.

26

The Fifth Time is a Charm

By Joanne Dalrymple

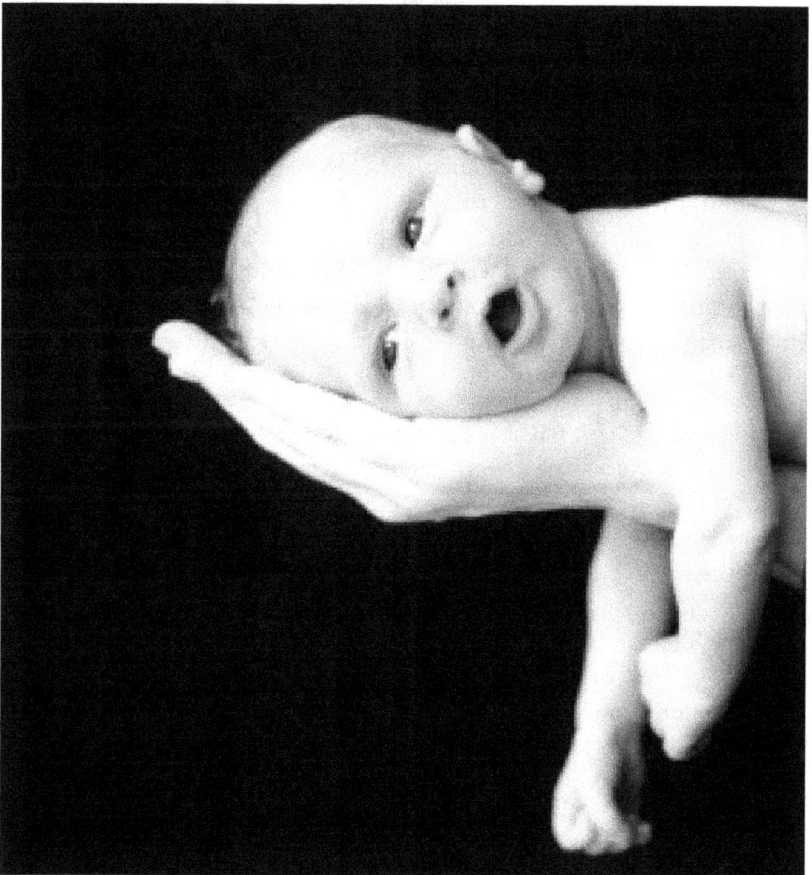

Murphy Dalrymple

As a young, first pregnancy mom, I thought the idea of a natural childbirth sounded great. I mean, I can probably count the number of Advil and Tylenol I've ever taken in my life. Really. I am not fond of taking medicine. Yet, I knew very little about the ins and outs of giving birth aside from what I had seen in movies and heard from acquaintances. I was the first of my good friends to have a baby. My mother had four children naturally and one with an epidural. She was indifferent about my birthing choices and said she'd support my decision either way.

The first time I was pregnant, my husband and I took the required Lamaze class at the hospital where we planned to birth and I read a couple of books about pregnancy, none of which told the wonderful benefits of a natural birth. My doctor said that it was pretty standard to get an epidural, but that some women chose not to. He was pretty indifferent as well.

I was so unprepared for my labor at 39 weeks. The contractions came much faster and harder than anyone, especially me, expected. I had to be put on medicine to slow things down because the baby's heart rate was decreasing. My body was convulsing, and when I was asked if I wanted an epidural, I said, "Yes! Right now!"

The epidural numbed me so much I couldn't feel my own breasts, so they shut it off. By the time I was ready to push, the epidural had worn off and I was able to push the baby out without any trouble, aside from the "needed" episiotomy, but I felt that I'd missed out on something. For hundreds of years women gave birth at home in their bedrooms in the most natural environment. Still, I didn't know how they did it after the pain I had experienced with the contractions.

Fast forward two and a half years. New state, new doctor, new everything. My second baby was nearly two pounds larger than the first, and at 41 weeks, still wasn't budging. Of course, the doctor wanted to induce me. So, at 41 weeks and one day, off I went to be artificially put into labor. My body actually reacted quite well to the Pitocin, thankfully. Now that I know more about Pitocin, I feel very fortunate. They were able to shut the drug off in less than an hour and my body took over. Everything went very well until the shakes, or as I call them "convulsions," started. Once again my body did not know what to do with this pain. I stopped progressing and once again opted for the epidural in hopes that it would relax me, so I would keep dilating.

Well, the epidural helped, but trouble was on the horizon. The pushing went well, the head was nearly out, and then the baby was stuck, really stuck, shoulder dystocia stuck. Out came the vacuum and a nurse running across the room threatening to pounce on me. I thought that this couldn't possibly be normal. This couldn't possibly be what God had intended when He created women for this very reason. However, we had a healthy baby girl and I rejoiced that all was okay.

Seventeen months later, I found myself in the same hospital gown, hooked up to the same dripping bag of Pitocin, thinking I was lucky that I had talked the doctor out of the C-section he wanted me to have because of the previous shoulder dystocia. My third labor was basically the same scenario as the second baby, without the vacuum and shoulder drama. The nurses couldn't believe how very little I needed of the medication or the fluid that goes along with the epidural. I realize now that I didn't need those interventions at all. I was much more in control of this third birth. We were blessed with another healthy baby girl, who weighed just one ounce less than our second.

Two years later, pregnant with baby number four, I was just as uneducated about natural birth as I was five years prior. At this point, I can remember telling people that my body just couldn't do it. I had convinced myself that my body would shut down from the pain and I was destined to stop progressing. Can you imagine? Boy, did I have a lot to learn!

Speaking of boys, we were going to have our first boy. I thought we'd do the same "drill" that I had become so familiar with. Although I still felt like I would have loved to have a natural birth, I somehow convinced myself that natural birth was just not going to happen for me and I needed to be okay with that.

My story gets very discouraging here. Same doctor, need I say more? The ultrasound showed a VERY big baby, and the doctor told us, and I quote, "I am scared to death to let you deliver vaginally. I mean, you've had three healthy babies … I don't think you should risk it."

Why, oh, why didn't I object? Well, maybe if I had I wouldn't be able to tell you about the most beautiful natural birth story, but I am getting to that soon. Anyway, his little speech was enough to scare me right onto the chopping block two hours later. Yes, you heard it here, after three vaginal births, I ended up with a C-section and it was horrifying. It smelled weird. I thought I had the shakes before?! During the C-section, I had the shakes while I was tied down. And are you ready for the kicker? The baby was not huge. He weighed just two ounces less than my second child who had the shoulder dystocia. That's one ounce less than my previous birth. I tried to make light of a very awkward situation and told the doctor to please keep sewing and not to put the baby back inside. Everyone laughed, but on the inside I was crying.

I knew nothing about C-sections. I had no idea the recovery would be the hardest thing I've ever endured. I had no idea I'd never fully regain feeling of my lower stomach ever again. I had no idea the scar tissue around the incision mark would still itch two and a half years later. The doctor told me this was good for me, and I believed him. "At least now you shouldn't have bladder problems later on in life," the doctor explained. *Really?!*

The light bulb finally, *finally* went on. Whew! I told myself if I ever got pregnant again, I was switching doctors and would search until I found one that would deliver me vaginally. I knew the previous doctor would not. He made it very clear that from here on out, if I were to have more children, they would be delivered via scheduled C-section.

Soon enough we had another positive pregnancy test. I made a phone call to an OBGYN office a friend from my church had recommended and I was on my way to a VBAC delivery. I finally decided to do some intense homework. I wanted to find out if VBAC was really the best thing for our baby, or was I just being selfish that I didn't want to be on the chopping block again? I spoke at great length to the obstetrician and sent out some e-mails to people I felt might know more about VBACs. It was unanimous— VBAC absolutely was the best thing for the baby and for me.

Still, I knew that I needed some encouragement. A very dear friend, Natasha Panzer, recommended a book by Ina May Gaskin. In it, Ina May explains the risks of Pitocin and epidurals when doing a VBAC. This was it. I was going to get my natural birth. Now, there was a lot of unconvincing I had to tell myself about my body reacting and progressing with dilation. I knew I needed more help. I remembered my friend Melissa saying she'd love to be a doula someday. She had had four natural births and the last one was a 12.3 pound baby. If Superwoman is real, Melissa is her! How could I ask for an epidural with someone like that in the room? One day, very early on in my pregnancy, I flat out said to her, "If you are really serious about this Doula thing, I need one and you probably need a guinea pig." She cried, signed up for the classes, and was the best thing that ever happened to my birth plan.

My pregnancy progressed and time was ticking. The doctors really wanted me to deliver on my own around 39 weeks because of the previous "baggage" I call it. Not only did I have the C-section to factor in, but the shoulder dystocia as well. I think Ina May would say that another dystocia was more of a risk factor than the VBAC.

No one was talking me out of this VBAC. A friend of mine, who is a NP in a NICU, e-mailed me with all the horrible possibilities that could happen, but I just knew in my heart that I needed to try. I tell you this because I really do believe that having a positive birth experience is at least 90% mental. If you put your mind to something and really, honestly believe you not only can do it, but will do it, then you will! There are risks for everything, as my OB said. Still, I tried to keep perspective in mind. There was a greater statistical risk of having trouble getting in my car and driving to my appointment than there was doing a VBAC. I think this was really important to keep things in perspective.

Thirty-nine weeks came and went. Thankfully, the doctors were very willing to let me continue with the pregnancy without induction. I really did not want Pitocin or breaking of my water. I was definitely my own advocate this time as well. I knew this baby wasn't as big as the previous three. (I was right, too. He was my second smallest baby.) I told my doctors this and said I was very comfortable continuing.

At 40 weeks and four days, the OB told me it was probably time to consider an induction. My heart sank, but only for a minute. I knew I just had to will this baby to come out before that date. So, we set everything up for five days from that day. It was Friday. I knew my favorite OB was on call three days later, Monday. I told my husband and my mom and anyone else that would listen that I would be having the baby with my favorite doctor on Monday. I contracted on and off all weekend long.

On Sunday night at 11:00 p.m., my husband called my parents to come over to watch our four sleeping children. He then called my doula and off we went to the hospital. I was checked in around midnight. The nurse checked me and said I was 6 cm and would be staying. I gave her my birth plan. The OB on-call said she was very comfortable with me staying off the monitor and not even prepping the heplock for an IV if an emergency arose. I said I was more comfortable being monitored and having the Heplock in place. I didn't think I needed to be too liberal. Even so, her confidence in me really helped. The doctor and nurse reviewed my birth plan and said it seemed like I really knew how I wanted this all to go and that they were just going to let me labor on my own with my husband and doula, and would only come in on occasion. Brilliant!

I, jokingly, okay I was serious, asked when my favorite doctor would be arriving. They told me he would arrive at 7:00 a.m. I told them we'd be having this baby shortly after that. They all giggled and said there was no way I'd hold out until then. Wanna make a bet? Remember what I said about mind over matter?

I labored through the night. My doula had me switch positions about every 30 minutes. At times, I really didn't want to move because I was comfortable, but this was something we discussed months beforehand. I knew it helped move the labor along if I didn't get stuck in one position. I anticipated being reluctant to move. She did a marvelous job of gently reminding me this was best for the baby. She and my husband made a magnificent team. They made me feel so special and strong. Melissa, at one point, asked, "How can you be laughing and cracking jokes right now? I was screaming my head off by this point in my labor." I don't know if she was telling the truth, but that was really encouraging and kept me believing that what I was doing was awesome. And it was!

I thought it was going to be so much more painful. It really wasn't. It was so empowering and natural. I truly felt like this was what my body was supposed to do.

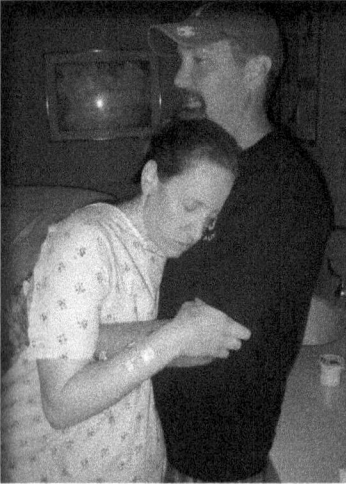

Joanne in transition

The nurse and doctor came in a few times. When I reached 9 cms, the nurse offered to break my water more than a few times to speed things up. I declined. I explained I really wanted this to be as natural as possible. Finally, my water broke on its own. It was the first time in five pregnancies and deliveries that I got to experience that! I was so thrilled. I remember saying, "So, my water really can break on its own!"

Throughout my pregnancy I read that it is helpful to have a focus object to help with pain management, but I just couldn't come up with anything. Some people liked to have pictures to look at, or there are other visualization techniques and such. Yet, nothing appealed to me. Finally, only a few days before the delivery, I found a Bible verse that spoke volumes to me. I thought if I needed something like that, this would probably be it. Well, during transition, I softly repeated the verse over and over, not even knowing until then that it would help, and focused on the number 33, which was printed on the corner of my husband's t-shirt.

I stared at the number throughout transition (good thing he wore that shirt I guess). I still couldn't believe how it didn't hurt the way I imagined it would.

The nurse was excellent about putting me into all different positions as well. She said some of the positions were really helpful in making the delivery much shorter. At 7:00 a.m. my favorite doctor entered. I sat straight up and exclaimed, "Praise the Lord! Okay, let's have a baby!"

Our sweet little boy was born at 7:41 a.m. The pushing was short and I welcomed it, as it felt like just the next natural thing to do. The doctor told me to stop pushing because he only had one glove on. I told him I'd waited all night for him to come deliver this baby, and there was no stopping now. He said he could catch him with one glove!

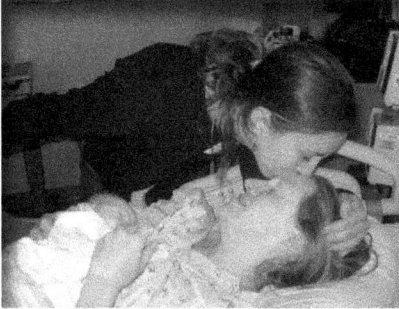

A kiss from her doula

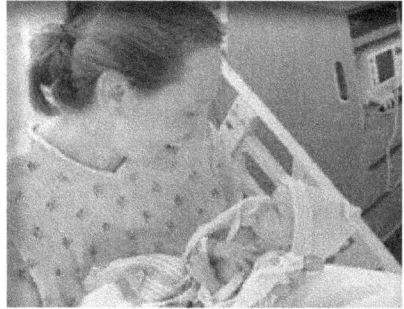

Joanne admiring Murphy

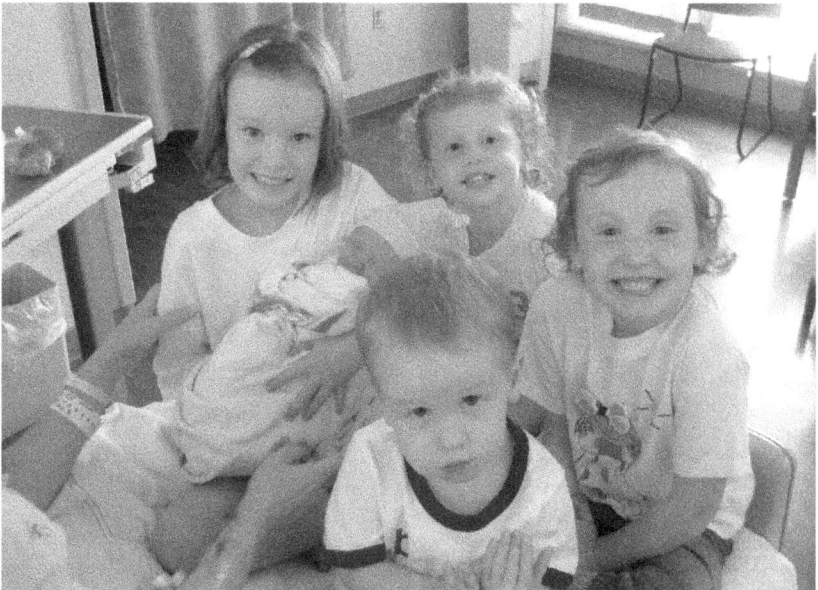

Riley, Abby, Molly, and Finley Dalrymple with baby Murphy

The entire experience was brilliant! I remember just minutes after our son was born, while snuggling him on my chest, announcing to the nurse, "Everyone should give birth this way! That was amazing!" And, "I wish I did this five children ago!"

I had a very small tear and the recovery was phenomenal. I was on my treadmill in less than two weeks. Yes, every mother should get to experience the birth of her child this way. And yes, the doctor got the other glove on in time.

Part V

Home Birth

27

Home Sweet Home Birth

Home birth is on the rise in the United States. In fact, between 2004 and 2008 home births have increased 20 percent (MacDorman, Declercq, & Mathews, 2011). No doubt the eye-opening documentary *The Business of Being Born*, produced by Ricki Lake and Abby Epstein in 2008, has continued to inspire many moms-to-be to stay out of hospitals and avoid unnecessary medical interventions. More and more women who desire to birth in the comfort of their homes are finding the courage and conviction to make their peaceful home births realities.

There are many advantages to birthing at home if natural birth is your intention. Home births, although controversial, are safe, providing the birth attendants are trained and competent. Women laboring and delivering at home will be able to have complete control over who attends their birth and, therefore, will be able to keep the atmosphere peaceful and comfortable—optimal for progressing steadily through the stages of labor. Home birth mamas will also benefit from the privacy and one-on-one attention. Opponents to home birth should know that the home is actually the safest of all environments in terms of infection, and most issues that arise can be resolved on site by a midwife, without transfer to a hospital (Goer, 1999). If you believe in your body's innate ability to birth naturally, are healthy, and experienced a normal pregnancy, home birth may be a very satisfying choice for you.

The following stories show the beauty and tranquility of birthing at home. The women who planned to birth in familiar surroundings did so mindfully, weighing the risks with the rewards.

28

My Fast, Easy, Pain - Free Home Birth

By Nancy Kelly

My due date came and went, but I wasn't upset, nor was I all that surprised. After all, my son was born 12 days past his estimated due date, and I expected to go past my due date in my second pregnancy, too. I kind of wished that this baby would come exactly 12 days "late" also, since that day would be my birthday—my 30th—and it would be the best gift ever. When that day came and went, my patience began to wear thin. How could my second baby come even later than my first? I was feeling huge, uncomfortable, and so ready to meet my baby.

I had been having Braxton Hicks contractions for weeks, if not months, but it wasn't until I was exactly 42 weeks pregnant that I began to have pressure waves (contractions) that I knew were the real thing. My sister and her husband were visiting us, and I told them I needed to go for a walk around the block because I needed to focus on the feelings I was having. I came back and told them that I was having sensations like the baby would be coming soon. By mid-afternoon, I was having one minor wave every hour or so. I was happy that my birthing time was coming soon.

I had been in close communication with my midwife, Christy, for a few weeks. Since I was getting well past my due date, she wanted me doing kick counts a couple times a day. On this day, my baby was not moving too much, and I called Christy to let her know. I told her I felt good about it, and that my gut instinct was that the baby was resting for the work that lay ahead. She thought I was probably right, but decided to come by that night to listen to the baby just to be on the safe side.

Once our midwife arrived, my husband, Chris, put our son Luke to bed while Christy listened to our baby's strong and happy heartbeat. After she left, both Chris and I began getting things in order for the birth. We had planned a home birth for our baby, and we knew that by the morning, our house would probably be buzzing with people and action.

My waves began to increase in length and intensity an hour or so before we went to bed. They were also getting closer together. I was no longer able to continue with my tasks during the waves, and that made me happy. The longer and stronger the waves, the closer I was to meeting my baby.

We finally went to bed around midnight, after a long conversation about baby names that ended unresolved. Although I was excited and couldn't stop thinking about the baby and names, whether the baby was a boy or a girl, and how and when he or she would arrive, I finally closed my eyes and drifted off. I awoke every half hour or so with the oncoming waves, and was able to drift back to sleep each time until about 3:00 a.m. At that point, the waves were about 20 minutes apart, and I thought I would be more comfortable in the bath. I didn't wake Chris, but went quietly to the bathroom with my iPod loaded with my Hypnobabies audio tracks to relax and gain focus on my birthing waves.

Despite my best efforts to relax and focus on the audio tracks, I was more focused on my phone, texting with Christy, and deciding whether to call my team. My team consisted of my mom, who would babysit Luke, my sister, Colleen, playing the role of doula, and my best friend, Becky, who also studied Hypnobabies in her pregnancy with her son and would attend this birth as photographer and gopher for whatever we needed. Ultimately, I decided to call my mom who had a 90-minute drive ahead of her and held off on the other two calls, knowing I had some time before they were really needed. Plus, it was still only about 3:45 a.m., and I wanted everyone to have some sleep since we didn't know how long they would be with us throughout the day.

Because I wasn't really focusing well in the bath, I decided to move to my birth ball. I found an extremely comfortable position, sitting on the ball, and leaning over the arm of our couch. I put on my Hypnobabies tracks while Chris filled the birth tub. He was also in charge of timing my waves. We discovered they were coming 8–10 minutes apart and lasted about a minute by about 4:30 a.m. I called my sister and Becky to come on over when they were ready. I also texted Christy with my update, and she said she would be with us soon. She called Janeyne, her assistant, to come soon as well.

Despite popular belief, I programmed myself to believe that pain was not a necessary part of the birth process. I used Hypnobabies to help me relax and focus, and to retrain my mind to know that birth was very natural. I managed to do this despite the fact that I had some painful sensations during my first birth. Somehow, I knew those feelings were due to the messages about birth popularized by media, TV, and movies. In this pregnancy, I was able to let go of all those negative messages and images, and focus solely on what birth was to me—a normal, natural process to bring my baby into the world. For each wave that came to me, I went inward and focused on what I knew to be true, and reminded myself that each pressure sensation I felt, no matter how intense, was not painful. During each wave, I reminded myself what my Hypnobabies tracks told me: that each wave was just a big warm hug bringing my baby closer and closer to me. So I really was comfortable, not only between the waves, but during them as well.

I spent about an hour alone on my birth ball until my team began to arrive. Once they were there, I was excited! It was nice to have some company in the early morning hours. We were kind of giddy, and we chatted happily between waves. In fact, once Christy arrived, she pulled me aside to ask if there was too much energy in the room. I assured her that I was fine and I was really enjoying the company and normalcy they offered. Since my Hypnobabies training advised that a calm and quiet environment would help me attain hypnosis, I was not surprised that Christy was curious about the buzzing atmosphere in my house. I think I was able to "go under" when a wave came upon me, and to immediately switch off and be "normal" when the wave was over. I think that's just my personality and how it worked for me, although I can understand some moms wanting a quiet, dim, and peaceful space for their birthing. Not so for me!

At about 7:00 a.m., Chris and I decided to take a walk around the block. It was still early, so we didn't run into any neighbors. We had to stop often for waves, and even though we had stopped timing them, I knew they were coming closer together and the intensity had definitely increased.

At this point, some women might have considered the waves painful, but my deep relaxation during the waves and my Hypnobabies practice helped me to identify the sensations as only pressure. The idea that these feelings were normal, natural, and positive overrode the desire to push them away. Somehow, even being outside with the possible presence of other people, I was able to completely tune out anything but my waves, and I relaxed completely during each one.

Upon arriving home, I had the one and only cervical check of my pregnancy and labor. Christy determined I was about 6–7 centimeters dilated. I think we were all a little surprised that I was so far along since I was still so "normal" at this point.

I credit Hypnobabies with helping me stay calm and focused, and to be in complete control of my sensations during waves. Because of my calm demeanor, it was difficult to tell how far along I was using behavioral cues.

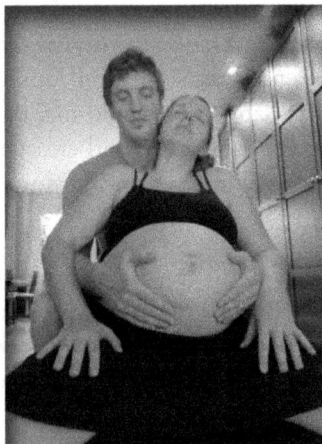

Nancy laboring on birth stool with her husband supporting her belly.
Photo courtesy of Christy Santoro, CPM, of Motherland Midwifery.

I tried to labor in the tub for about an hour, but to my surprise my waves slowed down, so Christy sent us on another walk. Within one minute of exiting the tub, the waves increased and intensified. Chris and I attempted a walk, but the waves were coming so fast and strong, we only got a quarter of the way around the block before turning back. It was about 10:00 a.m. at this point, and neighbors were out on this beautiful day; after all, it was Labor Day, and everyone was off from work enjoying the holiday. We ran into a few neighbors, who were very surprised to see me out walking during labor. We stopped and chatted with one friendly neighbor, but I needed to break the conversation for a moment to focus on a wave. We all kind of laughed that I went right back to our conversation after the wave was over.

Once we got back home, we decided to go to the tub again. I was so thankful for the relief the tub offered. It really cut the intensity of the waves, but this time, it did not slow the progress.

My whole team came with me to the tub, and Chris eventually got in with me to help me through the more intense surges. These waves were stronger, but I was still embracing them and letting my body do its work without interfering. I remained calm and never tensed my body during a wave. I knew that doing so would cause them to be

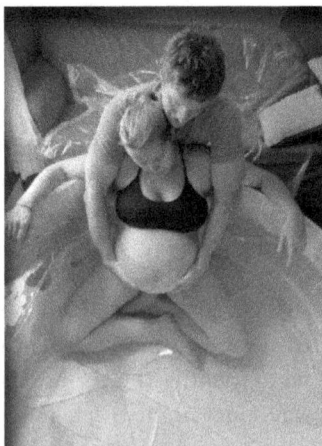

Nancy in birth tub
Photo courtesy of Christy Santoro, CPM, of Motherland Midwifery.

painful, rather than just intense pressure. While this was the most powerful part of the entire birthing time thus far, it seemed to pass by very quickly. What I remember most was the support of every person in the room. They were there to respond to my needs, no matter what they were. Even when the only thing I needed was for someone to crack a joke and help me laugh and smile a little, my team was there to help! I love each and every one of them for being there at such an important time for me.

I know I was in the tub for about two hours, but it felt so much shorter than that. It was some time around noon when I began to wonder if I should push. I did not want to push like I had with my son. With him, I held my breath and pushed so hard that I turned purple in my face, and actually burst blood vessels in my eyes. I had planned to just let my body do its job this time around, but my body wasn't doing anything different so far. I asked Becky to turn on the "Pushing Out Baby" Hypnobabies track. I guess I hoped that the messages in the track would help my body get into gear for the next phase.

Perhaps it was fate or just coincidence, but the next surge brought about a very different sensation. This time, it felt as though a gentle suction or vacuum was bringing the baby down even lower. I began to grunt involuntarily, and I announced, "I'm not doing that!" I know I sounded concerned, because everyone assured me what I was doing and feeling was completely normal and fine, but this was the first time in this birth that I felt out of control. My body took over, and I did not have to push. This must be what so many women had told me would happen: pushing would be an involuntary process, and I would not have to bear down intensely to bring my baby to me. My baby—and my body—did it on its own.

In the next surge, I felt like I wanted to help, so I pushed a little, and it felt so good! In fact, I remember thinking that I just wanted to help a little, so as to not overdo it like I had with my son. So mid-surge, I tried to stop pushing, only to discover that I could not. My body knew what to do, and was overriding my mental suggestions. Even at that moment, I remember thinking how incredible it was—our bodies are programmed to do what they need to do. And we are capable of doing this completely on our own! Remarkable!

At this point, I was still handling everything very well, but time seemed to pass so quickly. I felt the powerful force of my body bringing my baby further down. The pressure was more than intense, but still bearable.

After two waves, the baby's head was visible. After four waves, the head was out. During the fifth surge, our baby entered the world! Born in the water, in the sac, our baby joined our family peacefully, after a little gentle untangling in the loving hands of our midwife. Christy placed our baby on my chest, and we gazed at this baby that we loved so much already! The room was full of excitement and tears of joy. I couldn't stop staring at this baby, who also wanted to stare at me, too!

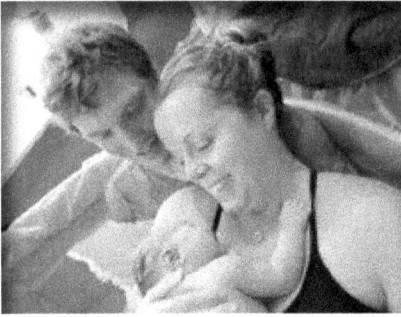

Nancy, Chris, and Maggie
Photo courtesy of Christy Santoro, CPM, of Motherland Midwifery.

After a few minutes, someone asked if the baby was a boy or girl. To my surprise, we still didn't know. Before the birth, I thought that I would want to know the gender immediately, but in the moment, it did not matter. Whatever this baby's gender, I was in love. I wanted Chris to be the first to know and to announce the big news, but he was behind me, so he had to reach around and feel whether our baby was a boy or girl. He whispered in my ear, "It's a girl... but I don't know if I missed something." So I looked myself to confirm, then proudly announced, "It's a girl!" I cried. A beautiful baby girl! We had not picked a name, but in our conversation the night before, Chris had a strong preference. When I saw our little girl, I knew who she was, so I whispered in Chris's ear that we should name her Margaret, which was his wish all along.

So there we were, in the tub with our baby girl. Christy wanted me to birth the placenta on the bed, so she could monitor my bleeding. It was only minutes after getting out of the tub and onto the bed before our little Margaret began to nurse happily and very efficiently for nearly an hour!

Christy has a practice of allowing the new family to bond for about an hour after birth, as long as mom and baby are healthy. Since all looked good with us, we spent that golden hour in our bed in awe that she had finally come. She was chubby and cute! We were in love and falling deeper with each passing minute. Maggie met her big brother, Luke, after he awoke from his nap just about half an hour after she was born. It was so wonderful for him to join us, even for a short while, during that special hour. It was beautiful to see him smile and want to kiss her right after he saw her for the first time.

After our special hour together, Christy checked me, while her assistant Janeyne began Maggie's newborn check. We both were doing very well, considering our recent hard work. We discovered Maggie weighed 9 pounds, 5 ounces, and I was uninjured and required no stitching at all.

After a trip to the bathroom and a super quick shower, Christy examined the placenta with all of us watching. She showed us both sides, and explained how each part works. We found out that despite being 15 days past our guess date, my placenta looked young and very healthy.

Christy and Janeyne packed up after a couple hours. They even showed us that they were leaving with two small trash bags, so we could see that home birth isn't as messy as most people think. I was so tired and couldn't be happier that my baby and I would get to nap in our own bed after everyone left. It was so nice to be home with the comforts of our own things and our own space around us.

So there I was, finally alone with my little girl Margaret, who we would come to call Maggie. Born a short nine hours after the beginning of our birthing time, born after a calm and pain-free labor, and born into our family in the water. It was a happy, calm, and wonderful home birth of a beautiful baby girl!

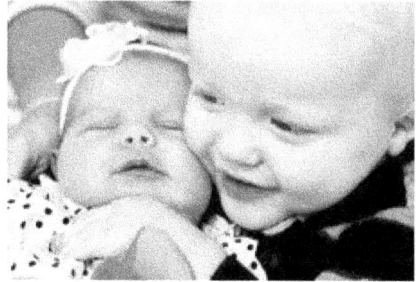

Luke and Maggie Kelly
Photo courtesy of Tricia Ebarvia
Photography.

29

Seren's Perfect Home Birth

By Amy Swagman

I think I knew I was going to be going into labor on Saturday night (May 22). I had just spent Friday and Saturday at the Colorado Midwives Association conference, listening to the legendary Ina May Gaskin. When I got home, I just felt like I needed to get the house ready. I was sort of irritable, flying around putting laundry away, etc. Kyle said, "Just do it tomorrow," but somehow I knew I should do it then. I had some sporadic contractions all Saturday evening (about 5–10 minutes apart, but nothing serious), then had a glass of wine and went to bed.

I continued to be awakened by contractions all night long, some of them even working their way into my dreams! I had a dream we got pulled over by two cop cars for making an illegal U-turn. I was in the driver's seat, but somehow Kyle was driving. They asked me to step out of the car and I proceeded to have a contraction (in the dream and in real life), and squatted next to the car. The cops sort of backed away and said, "Umm, never mind!"

I woke up around 7:00 a.m. with contractions that were about 10 minutes apart and 1.5 minutes long. They were stronger than they had been and just weren't going away. At that point I was thinking that I was maybe 75% sure I was going into labor. I got up to eat breakfast around 9:00, and as soon as I was upright, they got a lot closer together (three to five minutes), but still very manageable. I tried to eat some cereal, but was kind of nauseous and gave up.

Kyle took care of the girls while I spent some time in a lavender bath my friend, Ashley, had gotten me. The contractions would slow down to about 10 minutes apart when I was laying down, so I knew it was still early. I decided to take advantage of it and get some rest while I still could. I got out of the tub and laid down for about an hour. Haven came in to join me, and we cuddled, with her rubbing my back during my "belly squeezes." It helped so much to see her sweet little face looking at me during the contractions! I just kept thinking that I was about to have a sweet little girl just like the one in front of me.

I got up around 1:30 p.m. and Heather (one of my best friends) came over to hang out with our daughter, Haven, while our other daughter, Lyric, took a nap and Kyle and I walked around the park by our house. It was a BEAUTIFUL day! Blue skies, warm but not hot, light breeze, perfect. We had a leisurely time walking around, swaying during contractions and talking. We definitely got some looks from neighbors! The only down side was that there was only one port-a-potty in the park, and with Seren's head so low, I had to pee all the time. Whenever my bladder was full I'd have lots of contractions (about two minutes apart), which made walking to the potty really hard! Not to mention the ones I would have in the port-a-potty...

Stacie (my midwife) and Miranda (my friend and doula sister) kept telling me that I didn't have to keep walking if I didn't feel up to it, but it felt so good to be out in the sunshine. I even got a little bit of a sunburn during my labor, which I think is fabulous! We walked around for about two and a half hours, just making loops and walking with one foot on the curb when I could. Sometimes we'd sit for a bit in the shade and update our birth team. Heather was the only one at our house yet, so we were letting Stacie, Miranda, Jessica (our other midwife), Diane (one of my best friends), and Ashley (my friend and photographer) know where things were at in my labor. The contractions were (on average) three minutes apart while we were walking, and sometimes spaced out to five minutes apart when we were sitting down, so I knew we were down to business, but things were still early.

At about 4:30 p.m., I started to feel like we should head back to the house. We got home and ordered some sandwiches from Jimmy John's (the peppers were great until they weren't). I could feel something switching over in my mind and body, and I felt like I wanted to start turning inward and go inside myself. I sat on the couch, Lyric in my lap, and breathed through some strong contractions.

Stacie came at 5:30 p.m., and I could feel things starting to move into active labor as I sat rocking on the birth ball. The contractions were getting much more intense, much harder to relax into, and I started feeling sort of shaky. Stacie wanted to check me just once to try and figure out when to call Jessica, our second midwife. Seren's head was so low in my pelvis it was hard for her to feel behind it and all the way around my cervix, but she told me that I was safely 5 cm, if not 6 or 7. This made me so happy! I was so worried I'd be 2 cm and be disappointed. I told myself I'd be satisfied with 4 cm and happy with 5 cm, so this was perfect!

I decided I really wanted to get in the birth tub, and I wanted Jessica and Miranda to come. I wanted to give Jessica a lot of time since she was driving up from Colorado Springs just for us! I think everyone got here exactly when they were meant to, even Ashley who flew in from Oklahoma at 6:00 p.m. and still made the birth!

I got into the tub and have seriously never felt anything so wonderful!! The warm water washed over me, relaxing all the muscles that I could relax, and I felt like I could sink into the contractions so much easier! I labored in the tub while Jessica, Diane, and Miranda made their way here. Heather, Diane, and the kids played together outside, and it was fun to hear their voices in the backyard. I think it was a good distraction for Haven and Lyric to have some friends to play with them. They came up periodically. Haven was particularly interested and wanted to hold me through some "belly squeezes."

Lyric came up and saw me have a contraction on the toilet and looked a little concerned, but when she saw everyone's smiling faces (including mine), she seemed reassured.

I stayed in the tub most of the time, leaning on Kyle and moaning through contractions. Miranda was rubbing my back, and Stacie and Jessica would wipe my forehead and hold my hand if I needed them to. Everyone was perfectly in sync, and they were exactly what I needed! If one of them had to leave the room for something, it felt like there was a definite void.

The contractions were getting more intense and taking on a different quality. The contraction itself felt mostly muscular, but during the peak they started to take on a skeletal quality as well. My whole pelvis just felt sort of achy. This was different than my births with Haven and Lyric.

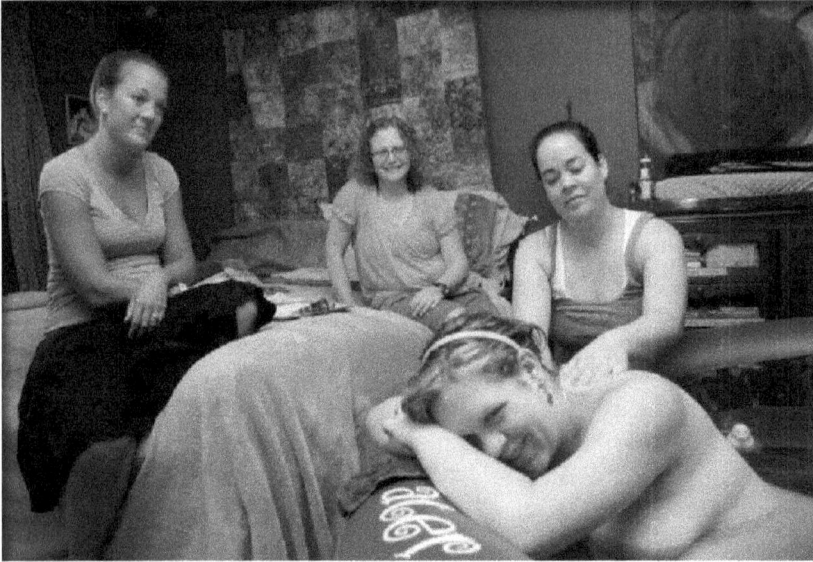

Amy in tub with birth team around her
Photo courtesy of Ashley Henry Photography.

It turns out that this was because Seren was facing sunny side up. For those of you who don't know, most babies come out OA (occiput anterior, or facing mom's back). If a baby is OP (occiput posterior, or facing mom's front), there is usually a greater surface area to the head, and the back of the head pushes into mom's sacrum causing what's called "back labor." Because I was carrying Seren totally different than Haven and Lyric (Seren's back was always on the right, the girls were always on the left), this was my number one fear! I've been at births with women experiencing back labor that described it like an axe embedded in their back, even in between contractions. It can also cause a lot of false starts to labor, long labors, long pushing stages, etc. I didn't want this to happen to me! The completely ironic thing was that I never had back labor.

Besides the sort of aching in my pelvis, it was completely normal! Not only that, but it was by far my fastest birth! Apparently, I have one of those pelvises that can accommodate an OP baby. Around 8:00 p.m. things started to get really intense. The contractions were coming about every three minutes, and it was getting more and more difficult to relax through them. In between, however, I was really able to relax and be present and happy about my baby being born that day. I asked to have some music played (Heart Sutra: Bliss and Serenity) and it just made me cry! It was the music that was playing at our wedding and at Lyric's birth, and it made me think of when my last sweet baby was born.

I was starting to think that this intensity was going to last forever. I had only been checked once (I had GBS, Group B strep, in my urine and everyone agreed on keeping vaginal exams to a minimum), and I had no idea how close I was to giving birth. I also had never lost any of my mucous plug or had any bloody show, the usual signs that you're getting closer. I was starting to think I couldn't do it. Jessica said, "Don't worry, she's just packing up her womb," which made me laugh.

And then everything happened at once, LITERALLY! I felt a huge gush as my water broke like a torrent. I immediately started projectile vomiting (on Kyle, sorry babe!), and as soon as that subsided, I felt her stretching my perineum. I shouted, "She's coming NOW, go get Haven!" That was all I could muster before my body took over and started to bear down. It was the most amazing, crazy, beautiful, frightening thing I've ever felt! Haven's pushing and birth had been very coached (first baby, epidural), and even though I waited for a while with Lyric, I never had that urge to push. This was completely different. My body took over and it was like I was hanging on by my fingernails! Jessica told me later, "It's like throwing up except it's throwing down," which is exactly how it felt! I'd never realized how strong the fetal ejection reflex is.

Kyle jumped in the tub to catch Seren like we planned (in his clothes, there was no time to put on a swimsuit) and Haven did as well. A few minutes later, Seren's head was born, it whipped around like a corkscrew, then shoulders, and then she was out. I couldn't believe how aware I was of every sensation. I could feel every contour of her body as she came out, and there was such a relief once she was out. I had really wanted not to tear with this one like I did with the others and had told everyone prenatally that I wanted reminders to go slowly, stretch, breathe her out, etc. Now everything was happening so fast that I felt like my mind was telling my body, "Slowly, breathe!" and my body was saying, "Nope, here we go, out she comes!" Even so, Stacie told me later that my body eased her out beautifully, that it took breaks when it should have to let her rotate, and that I stretched wonderfully. In fact, I didn't need stitches after all! I only had a "skid mark" that would heal if I rested enough postpartum.

From my water breaking to Seren coming out was just six MINUTES! At this point Lyric was upstairs as well. We had tried to get her up there for the birth, but everything happened so fast there just wasn't a good opportunity. She jumped in the tub with us and started blowing bubbles in the birth water (oh well)! The girls took turns smooching Seren's head and Lyric kept pointing to her saying, "Baby, nursing!" though quizzically looking at my empty belly.

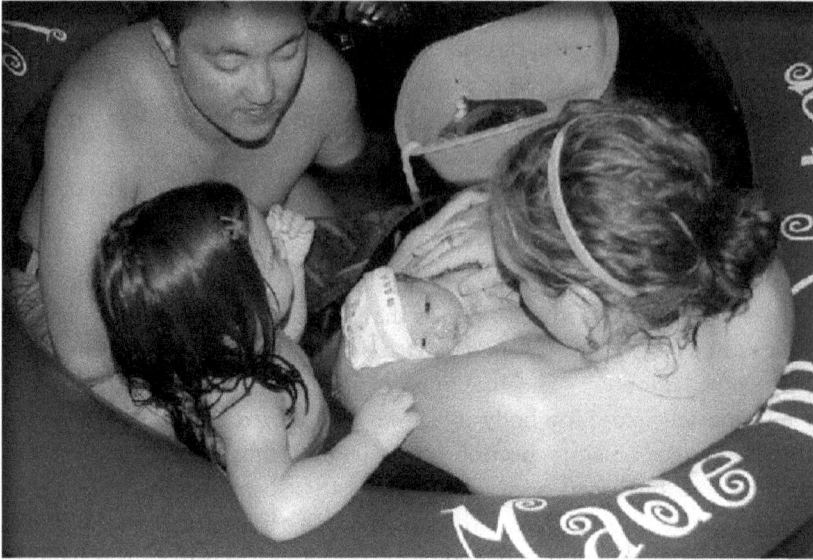

The rest of the family joins Amy in tub
Photo courtesy of Ashley Henry Photography.

We all looked our new baby over.

No one could get over the fact that she was such a pretty baby! So perfect and chubby, with a button nose, sweet little rosebud lips, and a little round head. She reminded me a lot of Haven, especially the nose.

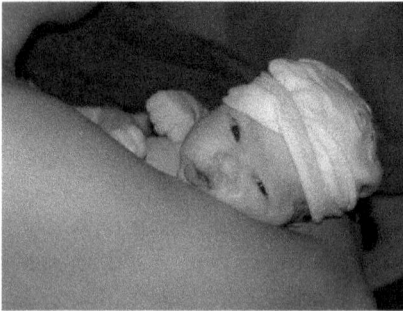

Seren
Photo courtesy of Ashley
Henry Photography.

Since she came out so fast, Seren was a little stunned. Her APGARs were 8–8 (off for color and tone), but her respirations and heart rate were as perfect as they had been during labor. A little postural drainage from Jessica helped her get some of the gunk out, and then she pinked up quite nicely (no bulb syringes at this birth, thank you very much!). Kyle felt that the cord was still pulsing, so we knew she was still getting lots of oxygen from the placenta. About 25 minutes later, Seren latched on (and I got a dose of Angelica herb). I felt cramping and pressure, as well as a little separation gush of blood, and then I pushed out the placenta. All in all, I only lost 250 cc's of blood, which is really great!

We decided to go and get cozy on the bed as a new family. Seren kept nursing like a champ. After a long while of that, I got up to try and pee, and

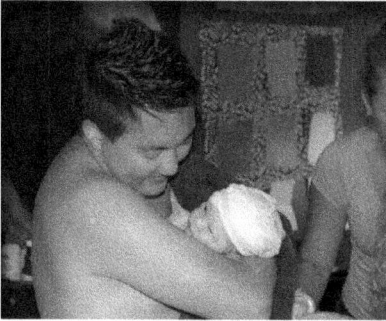

Daddy admiring Seren
Photo courtesy of Ashley Henry
Photography.

Kyle took Seren for a while. He was such a sweet daddy, smooching and loving on her. He had waited for a long time to hold an itty-bitty baby.

I came back and we did the newborn exam, and, of course, she was perfect, term, and healthy! Then Haven got to hold her (Kyle had to put Lyric to bed, she was so tired) and Miranda made placenta prints which turned out beautiful. I was feeling great, and Seren was nursing and pink and beautiful when everyone went home.

In fact, Seren nursed until 2:30 a.m. when I finally cut her off and gave her my pinkie finger, so I could get some sleep. She's still a champion nurser.

It was by far the most perfect, lovely, empowering, beautiful birth I could have ever hoped for! I absolutely loved giving birth in my own home because I could settle into my space and my body and it made everything really peaceful and manageable. I wouldn't do it any other way!

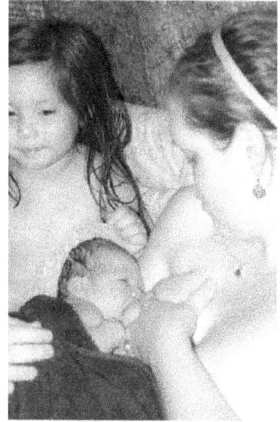

Seren nursing
Photo courtesy of Ashley
Henry Photography.

30

The Birth Dances of Eden Rose and Mica'el Sahar

By Jaquelin Levin-Zabare

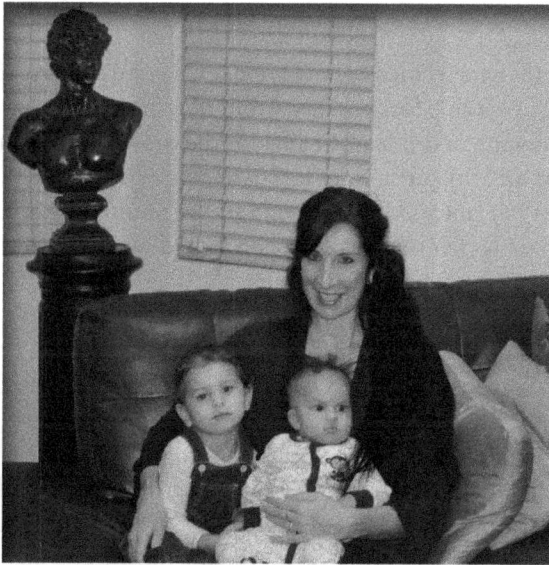

Jaquelin, Eden Rose, and Mica'el Sahar

I know that I had always dreamed of having a home birth when the time came to have children. However, I didn't realize it was a possibility until I did some investigation. While spending time and learning from some "sangomas" (South African shamans) in the rural region called Transkei in South Africa, I became so inspired by the matriarch of the clan, a woman in her late 20s, also a shaman, who had three small children. When I inquired where she had birthed her children, I was told that they had all been born in the very hut I was sitting in, as she squatted against the wall made of cow dung, straw, and mud, supported by other women in the community. Since then, whenever I thought about birth I would think of her.

I was born and raised in South Africa and spent many years traveling and living in different countries. I came to California by invitation to teach Vital Development Biodanza at the Esalen Institute, Big Sur. Many doors suddenly opened, and I was offered many opportunities for work. I kept on delaying my return flight to the UK, where I was living at that time. I was in Los Angeles when I met my future husband, fell deeply in love, and have never returned to the UK! We married in 2007. When I became pregnant in October 2007, I didn't realize I had any other option in the USA besides a hospital and Obstetrician/Gynecologist. As I was still new in town, I didn't have many friends or people I could turn to for some advice. I scoured the Internet looking for a female Obstetrician. I always preferred to go to female gynecologists, believing they would know how a woman experiences her body.

I found a doctor who seemed to have good reviews. At my first appointment, after being kept waiting for ages, I was told that the doctor shared a practice with a male doctor, and it was the luck of the draw who I would see at my appointments and my birth, if, in fact, a doctor would be there at all (at the appointments). If not, I would see one of the many nurses. I did not feel cared for. I actually felt that I was rushed in and out, and they had a whole waiting room of women to get through like an assembly line. The second time I went I felt worse. I had still not met any of the doctors in the practice. My husband and I were excited about this special time, and no one in that doctor's office made us feel special about it. As I was leaving this visit, the receptionist started rattling off a whole story about payments, blood tests, etc … a lot of information, and suddenly something happened that has never happened to me in my life, I fainted. I hit the ground with a thud and immediately became conscious of the sounds around me. The nurses and receptionist were panicking and called the doctor. I was lying down on the ground and he hovered above me. He said, "Do you know where you are?" I answered him and I heard him say, "She's okay," and then he walked off. My body gave me a strong message that day: get out of there.

As we conceived our baby in a conscious way, it was my intention to have the most conscious experience of pregnancy and birth. I set that intention and it seemed to get the ball rolling. I don't remember how, but I got hold of a book called *Beautiful, Bountiful and Blissful* by Gurmukh Khalsa. I was moved and inspired by her book, in which she mentioned home birth, and

I wanted to meet her. Many years ago I started practicing Kundalini Yoga and it transformed me by opening my heart and my life. Gurmukh is internationally renowned as a teacher of Kundalini Yoga. I went to Golden Bridge Yoga in Hollywood, California, and took a prenatal yoga class with Gurmukh. She has devoted herself to a path of helping people in many ways, from finding spiritual success in their careers and relationships to helping them consciously deliver healthy children and start their families off on a strong foundation. She is passionate, compassionate, wise, and wonderful.

It was amazing. I loved the wisdom Gurmukh imparted during class, and afterward went to chat with her. I asked her to recommend a midwife to me. Without even blinking, she said Davi Kaur Khalsa, who has over 20 years' experience as a Certified Nurse midwife in Los Angeles.

I went to meet Davi at her consulting rooms and immediately felt at home. The place was clean, pretty, and welcoming. It smelled good, with a candle burning and wonderful music playing. I was greeted and treated with such kindness. Davi came across so professionally. She made me feel that my pregnancy was a special time. She respected me and listened to all of my and my husband's questions and concerns. She took time to be with us, over an hour at each appointment. My husband and I were convinced that we had found the right path for us and the birth.

Birthing naturally was important to me because I believe in the instinctual and primal wisdom of the woman's body. My work in Biodanza Vital Development® (literally, "the dance of life") mirrors this belief. It is a unique system of human integration that uses music, movement, and emotion to re-establish an intimate connection with life. The system works by opening people's hearts and sense of joy, self-esteem, and self-confidence. It's simple, direct, immediate, and fun. This sense of joy and self-confidence carries over into people's daily lives. Over time, people find that life becomes more joyful. People start reaching for what feeds them in life and begin to change those things that are less positive. My work focuses on trusting that wisdom, about connecting to our deep sensuality and experiencing life from inhabiting ourselves completely. I prefer to heal holistically when I am out of balance, and I am wary of Western medicine—often used to numb the symptoms, but ignore the causes, despite the fact that my father is a doctor and my mother is a nurse. When I was about 16 years old, I made a decision that I wanted to experience as much as possible out of this wild, precious life, so I never had any fear about birthing. That was yet another experience I wanted to savor.

I was so blessed to be able to teach Biodanza Vital development on a regular basis during both of my pregnancies, and I feel this, along with prenatal Kundalini yoga, really helped to prepare my mind, body, and spirit for birth. I also walked regularly, as recommended by my midwife, Davi. She told me the yogis say that if you walk four miles every day, the baby will just fall out of you! During both pregnancies, I made a point of setting aside 20 minutes every day to meditate and visualize the birth. I also made sure I was conscious of my thoughts and feelings. I visualized the amniotic fluid crystal clear. This helped me to connect with my baby and establish a kind of dialogue with her. I enjoyed visualizing my baby forming healthfully cell-by-cell. Davi also recommended sitting in a sitz bath for 10 minutes a day to prepare the perineum and avoid tearing. I didn't tear with either birth.

Everyone was excited about the birth. For my parents, this would be their first grandchild, and they traveled all the way from South Africa to be with us for this auspicious event. My expected due date had been calculated as the 27th of June. It was a special time, and we spent some wonderful moments together before the birth traveling around Los Angeles. It was mid-summer and boiling hot, day and night.

My labor began about 24 hours before the birth. I started to feel twinges, but could still function normally. I had an appointment with Davi that day and she said I was in very early labor. I remember we were all in a deli eating lunch when the contractions started to intensify. I had to get up and walk around. I couldn't sit; it was too uncomfortable. When we got home, I spent some time in the outdoor spa with my husband and dad. I also walked around in the swimming pool. The contractions continued the same way, and I thought I ought to get some sleep.

I tried to fall asleep, but could not. I tried to relax myself by breathing long and deep, and I prayed for and visualized my baby safely being born. I communicated directly with my baby. At 1:30 a.m. on the 26th of June 2008, my water broke with a big burst and wet the bed. I woke my husband up to tell him and asked him to call Davi. Davi asked to speak to me and kept me on the phone for a while monitoring my contractions. I think she was deceived by my demeanor because I am quite a contained person. When I was having a contraction, it didn't seem so intense to her because of the way I expressed myself. Eventually, she said, "I'm coming. Lay down on the bed." I lay down and my mom was there rubbing my back. My husband was there, too, speaking gently and calmly, giving me ice chips and caressing me. I never felt afraid. I trusted in the Great Spirit and the intelligence of life and my baby. I remember focusing on a candle flame during my contractions, which were getting closer and closer together.

Davi had still not arrived. I felt a huge pressure in my rectum I knew to be my baby's head, and I said, "This baby is coming." I remained calm and focused on long, deep breathing and finding a rhythm within that. My mom and husband stayed close to me, but I knew that I was to cross this bridge alone.

Davi arrived and came upstairs to check me. She was flabbergasted to discover that the baby's head was right there. I couldn't hold our baby in any longer. She sent my parents to fetch her bag in her car. I asked if it was too late to get into the tub, where I had wanted to birth, and she said, "It is definitely too late to get into the tub."

She asked if I would be okay lying on my side. I said yes. I got onto my side and surrendered to my body's desire to push. As I pushed I could feel the movement of my baby further and further down. It was not painful; I just felt a lot of pressure. Davi told me to reach down and feel my baby's head. I think I pushed for less than five minutes, and my Eden Rose was born at 3:50 a.m. Davi caught her as she was chanting "wahe guru" (God is great). By the time my parents got back with Davi's bag, our baby had been born. Davi placed her immediately on my belly. I could feel the umbilical cord between my legs pulsating. I felt overwhelmed, elated. It took a while for me to connect the little being on belly with the sensations that had been inside my belly for the last nine months.

The birth of Eden Rose was a powerful and profound rite of passage for me. I always thought I knew about love, but with the birth of my Eden Rose, my heart opened up like never before. The birth was a beautiful experience. I feel that it was a shamanic experience for me in that it was so transformational. I learned about the strength I have within me and the power and wisdom of the female body. I feel like I entered into alignment with all the matriarchs of all the generations, and just like my ancestors, I had become a channel for life to enter through and part of the dance of life ripened and blossomed. The experience of the birth also enriched my relationship with my husband. We bonded stronger than ever before at the birth. He was an amazing support person and showed me so much love. My husband was deeply moved by the birth, too. We felt so blessed.

With my second pregnancy, I went straight back to our beloved Davi Khalsa. It was very challenging during this pregnancy to find time to myself, with a very energetic two-year-old. I was able to participate in few prenatal kundalini yoga classes at Golden Bridge, and then I also practiced at home when I could time, even if it meant my daughter jumping on my back and playing "horsey" as I did my "cat-cow" asana or my squats. I also taught my Vital Development Biodanza classes during this pregnancy. I walked a lot around the neighborhood with my daughter in her stroller. It was important to me to have at least 15 minutes a day to meditate and visualize my ideal birth and the healthy development of my baby. I made sure that I could have a few minutes each day to focus on and communicate directly with my baby.

My baby's expected due date was the 27th of August. That day came and went. At 42 weeks I started to feel a little nervous due to some scary birth stories I had read in pregnancy magazines. (Please avoid them!) Davi reassured me that all was okay and to trust that my baby would come when he or she was ready. She told me to walk five miles a day. I did that and continued to meditate and visualize the birth every day. A few days later, I started to feel contractions on a Saturday night. They seemed to stop and I was able to sleep. The next morning I didn't feel much happening, but they picked up later in the evening. After I put my daughter to sleep, I said to my husband, "This baby is coming soon. Call Davi."

Keeping my previous birth in mind, Davi didn't question me about contractions and got in the car to come to our house. We prepared the bed and I continued to move around and sway and slow dance. I couldn't sit down; it was too painful to sit. When Davi arrived I was leaning forward against my bed. I continued like this for a while, breathing and releasing each contraction with love. Davi's assistant, Nancy Beyda, arrived and asked if I would like a foot massage. I lay down on my bed and Nancy massaged me. She gently rubbed the soles of my feet first, then the tops of my feet and my legs. Her touch was calming and loving. My husband rubbed my thighs. It felt really good. Then I felt like getting into the tub. My husband prepared it for me and I got in. It gave me a lot of relief to be in the warm water. My husband was with me the whole time, feeding me ice chips, rubbing my back, and speaking gently to me. Davi and Nancy came in and out intermittently to check baby's heart rate and my blood pressure. I was trying different positions in the tub as the contractions intensified. I also vocalized from the depth of my belly in order to manage my contractions. I spent about three hours in the tub. Being in the water was relieving for a while. My contractions were getting stronger and closer together, and I felt a lot of pressure. There was a period of time when I felt so exhausted that in between contractions I felt myself drifting off. My husband was beside me the entire time. I was unable to find a comfortable position. I entered a space of silence, darkness, undulance. I could not answer my midwife when she spoke to me. I needed to focus deeply within, following the ebb and flow of my contractions and speaking to my baby, encouraging him or her to move downward. The pressure I was experiencing was intense. Suddenly, I felt a burst and my water broke. It was such a relief, and I started to feel so much better.

I felt myself entering a new phase of labor, and then knew I needed to stretch out my legs. I also wanted to stand up, be upright and walk around. Things seemed to happen quite quickly then. It was suddenly time to push and Davi asked what position I would like to be in for the birth. As much as I had wanted to birth in the tub, my body was now telling me I had to squat. My husband sat on the bed behind me and supported me as I squatted. I pushed for 10 minutes and my baby boy Mica'el Sahar was born at 1:10 a.m. on the 13th of September 2010.

I allowed myself to surrender even deeper with this birth. I wanted to draw on the primal energy to give me strength. I felt completely comfortable with my body and loved that I flowed with the sensations of the birth. I was able to be strong and vulnerable at the same time, and it felt raw and real and beautiful. I loved being in my peaceful home and feeling comfortable in an environment I could control. I loved everyone who was there and felt that we had all been on a wonderful journey together. I felt so strong, so beautiful, so alive, and thrilled with my femininity. This birth had been so different from my first birth, but just as amazing.

Davi's presence at both of the births was so special. I felt so safe with her and she really appreciates the sacredness of the experience. Both of my births were such incredibly positive and beautiful experiences that I decided I would like to support other women to have those positive experiences, too. That is why I have become a doula. Since attending births as a doula, both at home and in hospitals, my enthusiasm for natural home birth has been reaffirmed. Pregnancy and birth should be an opportunity for a woman to step into her own power. I believe that the wisdom lies in our bodies, and we need to trust our bodies, believe in birth, and trust the intelligence of the life force.

31

Conner's Birth Story: A Quick and Easy Home Water Birth

By Latia Murphy

At 9:00 p.m. on August 18th, 2003, I took 1 ounce of castor oil mixed with ice cream to make a shake and proceeded to talk to my friend Heather on the phone for an hour while I drank it. Contractions began immediately, and at 10:00 p.m., I finished up my shake, hung up the phone, took a hot shower, and then proceeded with an hour of breast stimulation, while rolling around and bouncing on my birth ball. I continued to have regular, painless contractions and ended up staying up to see if they would continue. I spent my time on my birth ball in front of the computer on my BabyCenter birth boards, and then wrote out a couple e-mails. At 2:30 a.m. the contractions were still painless and regular, so I decided to try and see if I could check my cervix to see if I was dilating and in actual labor. I went to the bathroom and when I sat down, I noticed some bloody show. Good sign, I thought, and knew I was probably in labor. I never even tried to check my cervix.

I decided to wake up my mom and tell her we should probably head to my grandma's house (where I had planned to have the baby) since bloody show meant I'd probably be having the baby within the next 24 hours. I told her there was no hurry—the contractions were regular, but painless. I got back on the computer, while my mom took a shower, to let the BabyCenter August 2003 moms know we were heading to my grandma's. I then packed my bags since I had planned to pack them during labor to kill time. At 4:30 a.m. we were finally ready to leave for the one-hour drive to my grandma's.

I called Didier, who was two hours away in Los Angeles, and told him to start heading to my grandma's, too. I then called my friend Amy, who was to videotape the birth, and told her I was leaving and would call her when I was in more active labor. Before we got in the car, I decided to time my contractions for the first time to get an idea of when to call my midwife. They were 1–1½ minutes apart and lasting 30–60 seconds! Wow! And they weren't painful at all. Maybe a little uncomfortable, like menstrual cramps, but that's it.

At 5:30 a.m. we arrived at my grandma's, and I proceeded to make the bed up, put out all the birthing supplies, and fill the inflatable tub with a little more air. The contractions were still just slightly uncomfortable, and I could still walk and talk through them just fine. After setting up the room, I decided to give my midwife a call and let her know I was at my grandma's and in early labor. I called her at 6:15 a.m. and left a message since she didn't answer her phone. As soon as I hung up the phone, the contractions hit hard and I had my first "painful" one. It kind of caught me off guard, and I ran into the bathroom and sat down on the toilet. The contraction had a grip on me and I started freaking out. I actually hit my head on the wall! I then told myself to calm down and got a hold of myself. I pictured myself when I used to run track, and just started breathing really hard and blowing the air out like I would do during my races. I sat in the little toilet room in complete darkness, breathing like this through each contraction. Finally, my mom and grandma started to wonder what happened to me and came looking for me. I yelled at my mom between contractions to fill up the birthing tub and told Didier to call all my friends who were supposed to be there for the birth.

I probably stayed in the bathroom for about 25 minutes, breathing through the contractions as I waited for the birthing pool to fill up. During that time I kept yelling to my mom to bring me water and Gatorade. I drank two bottles of water, a bottle of Gatorade, and then threw it all up. I got really hot and ripped off all my clothes, and then my whole body started shaking uncontrollably—I realized I was in transition! After what seemed like forever, but was probably only about 15 minutes, my midwife called back and talked to my grandma, who still didn't believe I was in labor. She just thought the castor oil had irritated my stomach. My midwife asked my grandma if my contractions were two minutes apart and all I could yell to my grandma was, "Yes, they're less," as I slammed the bathroom door. So my midwife said she'd be over.

Finally, after about 25 minutes of laboring in the dark bathroom, my mom said the birthing pool was about one third of the way full, and I immediately ran out and got in the warm water...Oh my God, I was in heaven. The water made the intensity 10 times less, and the contractions were so much more manageable. I didn't even have to breathe that hard through them anymore. I told myself I could labor in the water all day if I needed to. My mom had lit all my candles around the room and put on my relaxing classical music CD mixed with water sounds. It was so peaceful.

After I had been in the water about 10 minutes, my midwife and her assistant arrived and quietly set up all their supplies. My midwife had me get out of the water and on to the bed to check my cervix.

"You're complete with a bulging bag," she said!

I was in shock. She was in shock. We all were. Then I had a contraction while I was still on the bed lying down, and it was horrific. No wonder women get epidurals in the hospital—I would too if I had to labor lying down in bed the whole time! I jumped off that bed and back into my warm pool of water. As soon as I knelt back down in the tub, I felt a "pop," and I said, "My water broke!" Just then the baby's head slid down and was on my perineum. I could feel him coming out. I wasn't even pushing. I kept saying, "He's right there! He's right there!" over and over again. Then I reached down and could feel his head with my hand.

"He has hair!" I said.

During the next contraction, his head crowned, and I screamed during the "ring of fire." His head was out, but I didn't have an urge to push, so I waited for the next contraction, and then pushed his body out. The first thing out of my mouth was, "Wow, that was easy!"

Conner Piquet Murphy was born at 7:10 a.m., 55 minutes after my first painful contraction, and only 10 minutes after my midwife arrived. He was 7 lbs 15 oz, 21 inches long, and had a head full of jet-black hair. None of my friends made it to the birth on time, so we have no pictures or video from my labor and delivery. Even my grandma missed it. She decided to go to the grocery store to buy orange juice, and when she came back, my mom was holding my son!

I did end up tearing because it all happened so fast. I had a second-degree tear and seven stitches, but other than that, it couldn't have been any better. My midwife said it was the fastest first time delivery she had ever seen!

I've had many people tell me I was "lucky" to have such an easy and near perfect birth experience. I completely and 100% disagree. For nine months,

I worked extremely hard planning and preparing for my son's birth. From day one, I knew I would have home birth. My goal in life is to one day become a home birth midwife, and from my four years in nursing school, I knew that I did not want to give birth in a hospital setting. Everything I witnessed during my labor and delivery rotation in nursing school rubbed me the wrong way, and it was all just so impersonal and focused around what was easiest for the medical staff, not the birthing mother. I knew that unless there was some valid medical reason, the best place for me to give birth was at home. So at five weeks into my pregnancy, I found a home birth midwife whose personality clicked with mine and whose beliefs about the birthing process were in line with mine. Planning a home birth with a midwife I trusted, who I knew would be with me throughout my entire pregnancy and birth, was a huge peace of mind and totally took away any stress about not having my wishes followed during the birth process. I knew I wanted to be 100% present during my labor, focusing completely on giving birth, not fighting with hospital staff that I had never met and having to say "no" to every intervention they suggested. By planning a home birth, none of this stress would be an issue.

Besides planning a home birth, which is probably the most important factor of my amazing birth experience, I also worked hard to prepare my body for labor by eating extremely healthy and taking supplements known to ease labor. I followed the Brewer Diet and made sure to eat 80–100 grams of protein a day. This helps to prevent pre-eclampsia and premature birth. I took raspberry leaf capsules and drank raspberry leaf tea from five weeks into my pregnancy to two weeks postpartum. Raspberry leaf is one of the best pregnancy herbs and really helps to prepare and tone the uterus for labor. A toned uterus is more efficient during labor, making labor shorter and easier, and also preventing postpartum hemorrhage. I also made sure to take calcium and magnesium supplements throughout my pregnancy, as these supplements are also necessary for proper muscle function, and the uterus is a muscle that needs to be able to contract and relax properly. Magnesium is known to calm preterm contractions, as well as prevent leg cramps. I also took vitamin C since studies show that vitamin C decreases the chance of premature rupture of membranes. I wanted to make sure my bag of waters stayed intact for as long as possible since the contractions tend to be a lot stronger and more uncomfortable once your water breaks. Having an intact bag of water also decreases the chance of infection. All of these supplements helped to ensure that I remained low risk, which was necessary in order to have a home birth and necessary so that no time restraints would be placed on me (due to premature rupture of membranes or risk of infection). At the end of my pregnancy, I also took evening primrose oil, both orally and vaginally, to help soften my cervix, so it would dilate easily and faster once labor started.

I made sure to enroll in childbirth education classes that were geared towards having a natural birth, not a hospital or intervention-filled birth. I chose the Bradley Childbirth classes, which are a 12–week series that covers natural relaxation techniques, exercises to make sure baby is in the optimal position, the Brewer Diet, the stages of labor and the emotional signposts at each stage, pros and cons of all the routine interventions (and how to decline them!), creating a birth plan, hiring a doula, breastfeeding, and so much more. The classes are kept small, a maximum of eight couples, so it was an intimate class and I could ask questions freely. The Bradley Method is also great for the dads-to-be since they learn so much about supporting their partner during a natural birth. I knew that 90% of Bradley students who have vaginal births do so without any medication. I made sure to do my Bradley exercises (kegals, pelvic rocks, and tailor sitting) daily to make sure my baby was in the best position for birth and that my pelvic muscles were strong for pushing. The exercises help prevent a baby from being posterior since posterior babies often lead to longer and more difficult labors with lots of back pain. Posterior babies are also more likely to end up needing a C-section since they can be harder to push out if they don't turn during labor. The Bradley class really helped us to prepare physically and mentally to have a natural birth.

To make sure I was in the best possible mindset to give birth naturally, I read tons of natural birth stories and watched many natural birth videos. I also made sure to stay clear of the birth shows on television that tend to only show extremely medicalized births and births that follow the snowball effect–induction, epidural, C-section. I did not need scary hospital birth scenes in the back of my mind.

I read several books on natural birth, including *The Thinking Woman's Guide to a Better Birth, Ina May's Guide to Childbirth, Pregnancy, Childbirth, and the Newborn*, and *The Complete Book of Pregnancy and Childbirth*. I trusted my body and trusted myself to be able to birth naturally. I never had any doubts and was not afraid. Fear leads to tension, and tension leads to pain. During labor I followed my instincts and did whatever felt natural, whether that meant being alone in a dark bathroom, getting in the tub, or spending time on the birth ball. Laboring and birthing in warm water was amazing and really made the birthing process so much easier and more comfortable for me. I would definitely say that water is a must when it comes to birthing naturally.

All of my hard work seems to have paid off and definitely resulted in the most amazing birth experience that I could have ever asked for; an experience that has shaped who I am today and made me want to become a doula, so I can help other women experience what I did. As a doula I have now helped many women achieve the natural birth they wanted. I have since gone on and given birth to a second son, Parker Alexander Murphy, who was also born at home in the water in another near perfect (albeit slightly longer) birth experience!

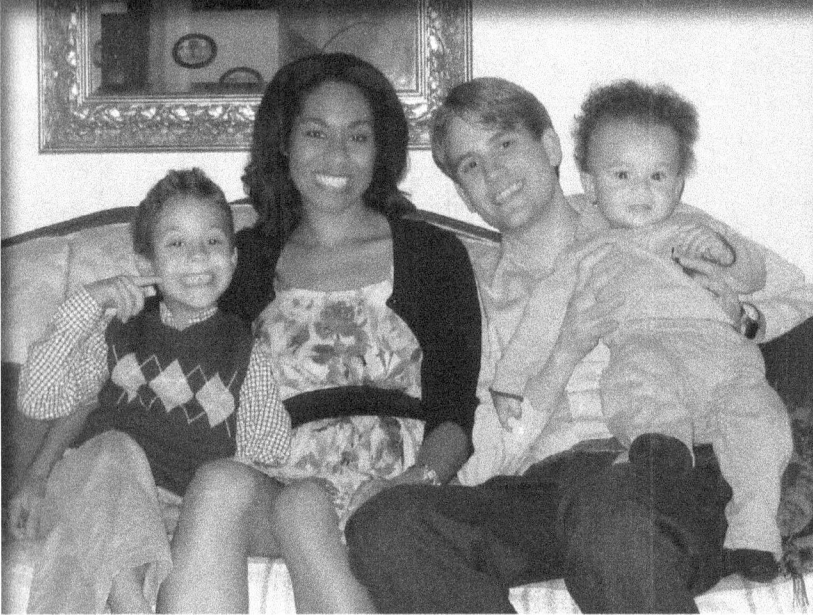

Connor, Latia, Didier and Parker

32

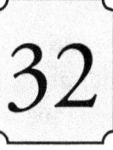

The Birth of Archer

By Janine Davis

This story comes to you from Bay of Islands, New Zealand

I planned my second pregnancy right down to the day; I even planned my honeymoon around the dates I would be ovulating, so that I would come home pregnant. Six pregnancy tests over the next ten days (I'm a little impatient) and, finally, a very faint second line appeared. My pregnancy was straightforward, a little uncomfortable, but I was carrying a very lively and healthy baby boy. His constant movement in the womb was definitely testament to his current personality, trust me my son can move...FAST!

After having a hospital birth in 2006 that strayed far away from my birth plan, I was determined to have a drug-free home birth the second time around. I stayed true to this plan until around 30 weeks when I started to freak out a little. The memories of my previous labor and birth began to come back and I began to question myself, "Can I really do this without an epidural?," "If I stay at home, then I really have to do it without drugs, I can't back out." Huge inner turmoil... I even started thinking, "Maybe if baby turns breech, then I won't have to do this, I'll have to have a C-section, and it will be out of my hands." This carried on for the next few weeks, talking myself into it and out of it. I finally came to the conclusion around 36 weeks that I was going to have my home birth. I had been so dissatisfied with my previous birth experience I needed to prove to myself that I was a strong and powerful woman, and my body was built to give birth!

 For the last 10 weeks of my pregnancy, I had almost constant Braxton Hicks contractions. There were many moments when I would think, "Maybe this is it?" Saturday night, sitting on the floor in front the fan (it was the middle of summer and humid), watching rugby with my husband, the contractions finally started gaining momentum. I say finally because the last few weeks always seem to drag and I feel like it's never going to really happen! A few hours later, things are heating up, contractions every three minutes, lasting for 60 seconds; I'm outside on the deck walking, swaying, leaning, and, most importantly, breathing! I decide to try and get some sleep in case I'm in for a long night. I sleep on and off for the a few hours, but labor always seems to intensify for me when I lie down. So I spend the night pacing the house, drinking tea, and gossiping with my mother-in-law. At 5:30 a.m., we call the midwife, and lo and behold, as soon as we hang up the phone, my contractions begin to weaken and become irregular. Umm déjà vu? I had a three-day latent phase with my first labor; I was devastated it was happening again!

Sunday carried on much the same way; contractions would become intense and regular for a few hours, then drift away. That night while trying once again to get some sleep, I spent the night on my hands and knees, rocking with every contraction. My husband woke up and rubbed my back each time, and fell asleep for the two minutes in between. I was up at 5:00 a.m. in tears and having a small tantrum, utterly drained, both physically and emotionally. A quick call to my midwife, and she arrived around 8:00 a.m. An internal examine showed I was 3 cm dilated, with bulging membranes. I sat back on the couch while my midwife did acupuncture, which calmed me down instantly. I went into an almost Zen-like state and felt invigorated and revitalized. I spent the rest of the morning in between contractions, preparing my room for the birth of my son.

By midday I was in active labor and my support crew had arrived. There were seven of them in total, my husband, mother-in-law, step-mum, best friend, two amazing midwives, and a midwifery student. I asked my midwife to rupture my membranes, as I was exhausted and very much ready for things to get moving. The next three hours were spent kneeling on the floor, laughing and talking, and leaning on the bed to breathe and rock

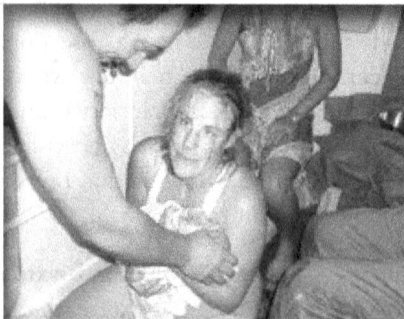

Janine holding Archer moments after the birth

through the now very intense contractions. My midwives were incredible, supportive, and encouraging. My step-mother, who had been a midwife, kept me focused on my breathing and put pressure on my forehead and the base of my head during my contractions. I had reggae and dub playing in the background, lavender oil burning, and my

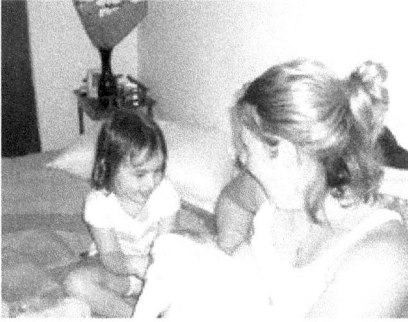

Ella-Rose watches as her brother Archer begins to nurse

husband massaging my back through every contraction. He did not leave my side once during these intense hours; I drew so much strength from him and his calm, quiet presence.

When transition hit, I was completely unprepared. I missed it the first time around due to the epidural. I will be completely honest with you—transition is hard! I felt emotional, scared, and in a lot of pain. I actually decided that I had had enough and stormed out of the room, as if I could escape it! Next thing you know I'm sitting on the toilet, refusing to carry on, and my midwife announces I'm fully dilated and ready to push. Thethought of walking back to my room was too much to bear, so I got on my hands and knees and pushed, 15 intense minutes later, Archer Riley Davis was in my arms, 7lb 11oz of perfect baby boy! WOW!!

I waddled back down the hall to my room, lay in bed, and breastfed my wee man within minutes of his birth. It was perfect. I was in my home surrounded by people who loved me, lying in my own bed, feeding my perfect wee son, with my daughter admiring her baby brother.

To top it all off, I had never felt so empowered. I was on a high! I WAS a strong powerful woman; I had brought forth new life without pain relief and medical intervention. I was proud. I was fulfilled. I had a son. Bliss.

33

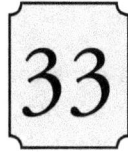

My Birth Experiences

By Susie Sams

Note: The home birth of Naomi Aroha Sams took place in New Zealand, the Sams family currently resides in the United States.

My first child was born in a hospital under the supervision of an OB/GYN. I had always dreamed of having a home birth, but I was recently married, young, and uninformed. Our apartment was the size of a shoebox—too small I was sure for a home birth. So I decided for my "first round," I should probably just go to the hospital to be "safe."

I was 38 weeks pregnant when I broke out in hives all over my belly, buttocks, and thighs. I itched and scratched 24 hours a day and was completely miserable. I had no idea what, if anything, was safe to take, so I just suffered through it.

When I visited my OB in my 39th week, I was told the only way for it to go away (diagnosed P.U.P.P rash) was to induce my labor. I was scheduled to go in the following morning at 39 weeks, 1 day.

The next morning, April 11, 2006, I arrived at the hospital with my husband. We were processed in, through mountains of paperwork, and they explained how they would start my labor. They began an IV drip of Pitocin and broke my waters with a plastic hook. I remember the hook hurt quite badly, and I could see the doctor was pushing very hard. My daughter was born four hours later, after a quick and intense birth, complete with an unnecessary episiotomy that required 30 stitches to close. I had taken a dose of IV drugs—Nubain, that made me feel so loopy and out of it that I heard crickets in my room when there were none. I consented to the episiotomy under the influence of Nubain, a choice I'd told myself beforehand I would not make. She had scrapes all over the top of her head from the hook. Oceana Faith was 7 lbs, 11.5 oz and 20 inches long.

When I became pregnant with my second child, I did a lot of research, because I had not enjoyed my hospital birth. The episiotomy had left scarring on my perineum and I wanted desperately to evade another cut and stitches. At 20 weeks we were told my son had a neural tube defect called an occipital encephalocele and would most likely be stillborn or die within hours of birth. He was born in a New Zealand hospital, under the supervision of doctor and two midwives. My labor was induced, but I was able to labor without any drugs or an epidural.

Joshua Matthew was 6 lbs 8 oz and 17 inches long. He was born alive and lived at home with us, for 69 unprecedented days. His birth was beautiful— quiet, calm, and joyful—despite the fear we had that he would not even be born alive.

My third pregnancy was a bit rockier. Because of our previous experience with Joshua, I spent a lot of time worrying about this new baby. I connected with an amazing midwife who helped me take the supplements I needed and gave me access to additional testing to set my mind to rest (extra blood work and ultrasounds).

On Tuesday (7th) my due date, my midwife and her assistant, a student midwife, came to the house to see me. Shirley (the midwife) did a stretch and sweep (stretching the cervix and separating the membranes inside the cervix) and I felt crampy and gross for the rest of the afternoon. I had some contractions overnight, but they were 20 minutes apart, and I slept through most of them.

I felt fine Wednesday (8th) and went out for the morning. I took a big walk with Oceana, and then came home. I lost bits of mucus plug all day. Again, I felt crampy and gross all day, but the contractions were not regular.

Thursday morning (9th), I felt fine again. I went out to lunch with my sister and took another walk. From 2:00 p.m. that day, I had contractions around 10–20 minutes apart, but they were still sporadic and not very strong. They were no more intense than on the previous days. I timed them before bed at 10 minutes apart, but still not stronger.

I sent Shirley a text message to warn her I might call in the night. I woke up at 4:00 a.m. angry that I wasn't in labor, but I was still contracting. I couldn't sleep, so I got up and had a bloody show, and lost more of my mucous plug.

I tried to sleep, but the contractions were coming regularly at 8–10 minutes and getting stronger. I dozed restlessly until 6:00 a.m. The pain was picking up. Because I didn't want Oceana (three years of age) getting scared that I was in pain, I had my sister drop her off at my mom's on the way to work (7:30 a.m.). The last half hour before Oceana left I was turning my face into pillows or pulling my sweatshirt hood over my face, so she wouldn't worry about me. I had lost my ability to labor without showing it in my face. She's very sensitive to other people's pain and I didn't want her to start crying about my scrunched-up face.

I labored on the living room couch for about an hour, and then finally called Shirley to see if I was far enough along. I doubted myself a lot because my two previous births had been induced when I was having no contractions.

My contractions were still slightly sporadic, varying between four to eight minutes apart, but never more than eight. I began to clean and do laundry; I felt quite a drive to have this tidy and clean house at this point.

Shirley came by 9:00 a.m. and started me on a homeopathic remedy to regulate the contractions and soften my cervix. The remedies were cauldophyllum to regulate my contractions and gepsemium three to four times to ripen my cervix. They worked! I found out the next day the cauldophyllum was specifically for regulating contractions during occiput posterior labor (sunny side up). Shirley knew I had been worried about a posterior labor, and that if she told me, I would fixate on the issue. So she never told me until everything was over.

I labored on my yoga ball, kneeling on floor and leaning over it. It worked great for letting me roll my hips without having to be on my feet. I laid or sat on the floor between contractions. Matt was watching the Master's Cup on the internet; we said maybe this baby will be his little golfer and Matt could be her caddy.

The student midwife, Shona, also arrived, and the three of them (Shirley, Matt, and Shona) hung out. They did some dishes, made coffee, and did paperwork while they waited for me. After a while they decided it was time to get their stuff sorted out and asked where I wanted to birth. I said probably upstairs in our bed. They went up to prepare and very quickly came back downstairs and pointed out that I might not want to go up the stairs while in labor, and since the bathroom was on our first floor, perhaps I would prefer to birth in our living room. So instead they pulled my sister's mattress off her bed, and put it in the middle of the living room floor.

I moved onto the mattress. They wedged the yoga ball at the end of the bed, so I could be comfy while hugging the ball. My knees were beginning to hurt from kneeling on the carpet. It was at this point that I started moaning through most of the contractions.

I could not find a position that was comfortable anymore. I had been on my knees, draped over the ball, but also tried sitting and lying on my left side. Left side was okay, but I felt out of control. I must have been in transition at this point, but it was different than my other two, so I didn't realize what was happening. I thought I had a while left to go when Shirley started telling me that I could probably push a bit if I felt the need. I was confused because I didn't feel pushy at all. She had a look, but no internal exam and said she could see the head. Again, I was shocked, as I didn't feel they baby's head yet. Turned out she saw a clot passing and felt bad for throwing me off when she realized it later.

A few minutes later she did an internal exam. She told me that I needed to wait a bit because I was at 9.5 cm, with an anterior lip. She tried stretching the last bit out over baby's head. She said she felt the baby's head turning into position just as she did the exam. Pretty soon after that I had a contraction (had been on left side), sat bolt upright, and flipped over onto my hands and knees. I started pushing gently. I felt like I was "testing it out" to see if I actually did need to push. I had a small trickle of amniotic fluid, and they checked to confirm that's what it was, but 10 minutes later my waters really broke. My midwife Shirley was in the way, but she just laughed and said something about getting a shower later. I birthed half sitting/half lying on my left side. My pushing wasn't regulated or "ordered." Shirley and Shona just had to keep reminding me to push with my chin down, not lolling back. It was probably only three or four pushes, as it was only 15 minutes from water breaking to holding my baby. Her head came out and she started to cry. One more push and she arrived at 11:55 a.m. on 10 April 2009.

Shirley made a point to say very quickly, "WOW, she's big!" Shirley had guessed that she weighed around 6 pounds. Instead, she was my largest baby at 8 lbs 2 oz and 20.5 inches long. I had no tearing or stitches, which was such a relief to me.

I spent my next few days, wrapped up on my couch holding my new baby girl. I felt comfortable and unrestrained. Naomi's labor and birth is one of my sweetest memories.

Naomi Aroha (Meaning: My pleasant delight, my love) 8 lbs 2 oz, 20.5 inches long Born 11:55 a.m. on 10 April 2009 (New Zealand time) She had a little bit of dark blonde hair and dark slate gray/blue eyes. Her chubby cheeks looked just like her sister's, and right away she had an attachment to sucking her thumbs and hands. Today she is a busy little girl who talks up a storm. I am truly blessed.

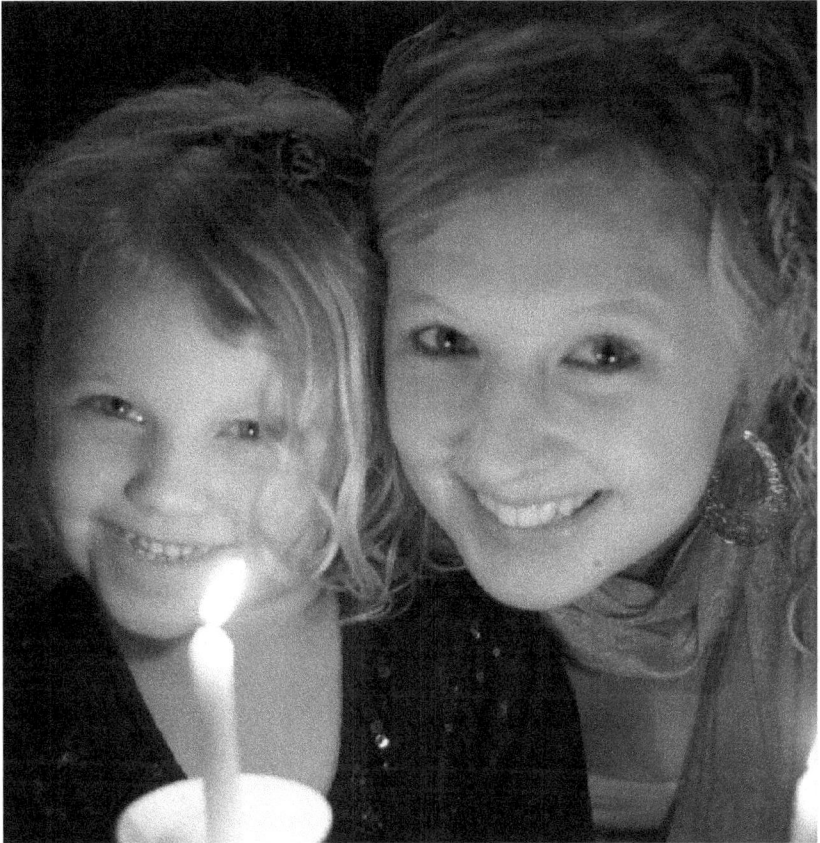

Susie and Naomi

Part VI

Unexpected Home Births

34

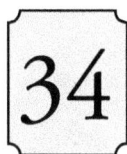

Calm Under Pressure

The final stories I chose to include in this collection show how incredibly satisfying birth can be, even when it strays far from our plans. When their labors progressed unexpectedly quickly, they let instinct be their guides and the following three mothers took matters into their own hands, bringing their eager babies safely into the world without midwives, doulas, or doctors. With quick thinking, calm, and grace (and some assistance from their husbands), they delivered their babies in their own homes. These births might not have been anything close to what the parents had planned for, but they were immeasurably empowering.

35

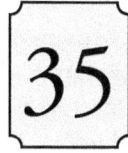

A Blissful Storm

By Viviane Elliott

Some of my fondest memories as a child are of visiting Switzerland with my family every summer. My mother was born and raised in the mountains of the Jura region, and during our visits, she would always point out a small chalet nestled away in the tiny village of Courrendlin. It was in this modest little chalet that she was born, and her aunt, also the village's midwife, delivered my beloved mother and her five siblings into this world. For as long as I can remember, my belief in natural childbirth began with this enchanting fairy tale image and developed into an intellectual and spiritual belief that as a woman, this is what my body is meant to do.

Yet somewhere towards the end of my first pregnancy, I lost sight of this vision. I became fearful of something I was passionate about and began to dread my upcoming delivery. Perhaps it was the tour of the labor and delivery unit where I planned to deliver that ignited such unexpected feelings of anxiety and insecurity. Forceps, vacuums, internal monitors … all of the 'worst case scenarios' were presented to us with pride that this facility could handle any emergency. Who wouldn't begin to doubt their natural ability to cope with childbirth after that tour?

The birth of Ciela, my first child, became a series of medical interventions. I had a difficult, but cherished pregnancy, and in the end, no amount of 'birth planning' would have been enough to prepare me for the invasion of interventions the doctor on-call insisted upon. I was first told that my baby was too big, and if I didn't opt for induced labor, then I was looking at a high chance of a C-section (a "50 percent" chance, according to the doctor, based solely on my size). Unfortunately, I did not educate myself enough to stand up for what I knew would be a natural process. I put my trust in my obstetrician and let go of my plan for a drug-free and peaceful birth.

My induction was relatively fast, extremely painful, and incredibly stressful. I was started with Cytotec to ripen my cervix and a Foley catheter to help dilate me to four centimeters. Once the Foley balloon fell out, Pitocin was started. I ended up with an epidural, a doctor who wanted nothing more than to cut me open so he could go back to sleep, and an episiotomy. I gave birth to my daughter lying flat on my back staring up at fluorescent lights. However, I was very fortunate that my nurse was a midwifery student and was a huge advocate for me during labor. She knew how important a vaginal birth was to me. And throughout all the pain of my Pitocin laden contractions, I can still remember her arguing with the obstetrician, "Just give her a chance! She can do this." With a threatened emergency C-section looming over our heads, Ciela's arrival into this world was a race to the finish line as opposed to a beautiful journey. Although her birth was indeed joyous, I cannot even begin to describe the relief Scott (my husband) and I felt as soon as she made her entrance.

From the moment I found out I was pregnant with my second child, I knew that everything about the upcoming birth would be different. I owed it to myself, and most of all to my baby, to experience a birth the way nature intended. This pregnancy was a second chance to find my voice and to let my body handle what it was designed to do. Although I did see an obstetrician for a large portion of my prenatal care, I made the decision early on that I would switch to a midwifery practice when I hit 32 weeks. I also hired a doula knowing that any extra support I could get would help me achieve my goal of a natural birth.

My biggest hurdle the second time around was that I was so traumatized by my first labor and delivery. Drugs, hospital lights, and fear had become the image of what delivering a baby was to me. On top of that, I completely doubted my tolerance for pain. What I didn't realize was that I had never experienced so much as a contraction without the use of a Pitocin drip.

I ultimately chose a practice that delivers in a hospital about 25 minutes north of where we live. I was too nervous to try a birth center because I didn't trust myself enough to not have the option of drugs. However, this hospital had birthing tubs, was very pro-breastfeeding, and promoted as natural an experience as possible, despite being a traditional hospital setting. Despite all of this, the self-doubt still lingered and I feared the upcoming birth of my son instead of welcoming it.

When I was 18 weeks pregnant, everything in my world turned upside down. It was the darkest time of my life; a time so painful that everything just seems a blur. My mother died. My mom was everything to me, and my biggest comfort in this world. She was the one who understood me the most. She was gone and I was broken. I made myself forget about my pregnancy. I guess this was my coping mechanism, my means for survival. I couldn't bear to think about this new life growing inside of me, as I knew my mother would never meet my baby.

However, despite everything about this despairing time, my perspective changed on so many levels. All my prior fears about birth seemed so trivial after I had watched my mother in sheer agony. The mourning that I experienced after such a loss was more painful than anything else I could fathom. Birth seemed like nothing to me. Are you kidding? I would birth a hundred babies in a row, drug-free and strapped to a table if it could bring my mom back to me. I toughened up in a way I never really wanted to, but I knew after the emotional trauma my family had endured, that I could handle anything.

I had my last midwife appointment when I was exactly 40 weeks along. She did a cervical check and determined that I was about one centimeter dilated, but felt that was probably only because I had already had a baby. I was told not to be discouraged and I wasn't. I always assumed that I would go late, and with the support from my midwives and doula, I knew that I would go into labor when my body and my baby were good and ready.

To my great surprise, I began having some bloody show late the next evening. I was thrilled that my body was starting to show signs of readiness and that I would probably go into labor on my own. I figured that now might be the time to put together that mix of songs for birth. My lavender oil was packed, as were some pictures of my mom. These items were to bring me encouragement and inspiration.

I went to bed past midnight, but couldn't sleep because I was getting so excited and also a bit nervous. It was lying in bed that I realized I was having some minor cramping. It felt like menstrual cramps, but my mind was going a mile a minute, so I figured that sleep was just not going to happen. I got up, packed Ciela's bag for her upcoming stay with my sister, wrapped a birthday present for the party she was going to the next morning, and just milled about the house. Ciela woke due to all of my milling and Scott thought it was best that we just call my sister to come get her. After all, we would probably end up heading out to the hospital in the morning, so why not have one less thing to worry about?

I was instructed by my midwife and doula to labor at home for as long as possible. "You will know when to come in," they had said. "When you can no longer talk through contractions, you'll just know." Well, I felt pretty good, so I figured I had a long road ahead of me.

At around 3:00 a.m., my sister came to pick up Ciela, who couldn't have been more excited to go have a sleepover with her auntie. I was starting to have contractions at this point, so I called my doula to let her know that I was pretty sure labor was starting. She seemed pleased and asked if I wanted her to come over. I told her it was nothing I couldn't handle and I would keep her updated. Remembering a documentary I had watched in which a woman kept going about her daily routine while in labor, I sat down to eat a big plate of scrambled eggs before I settled into the tub.

Labor was definitely starting to pick up at this point, so Scott and I began to time contractions. They seemed frequent enough, but weren't very long. Yet I was starting to get a bit uncomfortable. The alternation of the hot shower hitting my back and soaking in the tub provided a huge relief. Regardless, Scott was pressing for me to call my midwife and let her know what was going on.

My cell phone recorded the time of my call to the nurse on duty as 3:41 a.m. It was Maria who was on call and I was thrilled. I had been hoping all along that she would deliver my baby boy and what luck! We chatted for a bit. She asked me to refresh her memory about my previous birth, and I kept having contractions while on the phone. She said that since it was my second baby and I was Group B Strep positive, I should come in and get checked. With the Strep, I was supposed to have IV antibiotics administered every four hours during labor. The worst that would happen, she said, was that they would send me back home to keep laboring.

However, as soon as I hung up the phone and stood up from out of the tub, my whole rhythm changed. Contractions went from manageable to completely on top of one another. I figured that I had just hit active labor and perhaps I was now four centimeters dilated. I started yelling to Scott to pack me a water bottle and get my clothes. My mind seemed to go somewhere else and I just started aimlessly running around the house. At one point I remember flinging myself on the bed with Scott trying to get some pants on me. The pants were too much effort, so the t-shirt I was wearing had to suffice.

I had a flash of panic, a complete moment of weakness, where I knew that as soon as I reached the hospital I would demand an epidural. The whole process at this point was intense and the thought of five, eight, 12 more hours of this was unbearable. I dreaded every bit of this birth and thought to myself how crazy I was to think I could do this naturally. If I felt like this in early labor, how could I possibly manage the intensity of transition?

Scott was doing his best to get me out the door. We made it to the living room, about a foot and a half away from the front door. I couldn't bear the thought of a car ride right now. I needed space and to be able to move. There was crying, there was pleading, and there was a lot of screaming. Scott was on the phone with my doula at this point, who had called to check in. When she heard all the commotion I was making, she told him he needed to call 911. She had gotten to know me well during my pregnancy and knew that my tirades were not one of an overly dramatic woman.

And then, there was what seemed like an explosion. "My water just broke!" I screamed while falling onto my hands and knees. I reached down and couldn't believe it, "Oh my God, I feel the head!" It was then that I realized I was having this baby right then and there. Normally, one would think this would be terrifying. However, I immediately felt this huge sense of relief and knew with everything in me, that things were going to be fine. It was such a moment of serenity in this storm. I was birthing this baby on my living room floor and my husband was going to have to be my midwife.

Scott had called 911 only to hang up on them. I don't think he fully understood what was going on or maybe he just needed some extra time to process everything. He was still trying to persuade me to get up, so we could get to the hospital. 911 called back and asked if everything was all right. "Umm, I think my wife is in labor," Scott said. They asked if we were going to the hospital and if things were okay. He then looked over at me, took a closer look, and I remember hearing, "Holy sh*t, I see the head!" at which point he hung up on them again.

I was still on my hands and knees and my body started doing exactly what it needed to do. It was as if I surrendered and let this overwhelming force take control. I began to push a few times. It felt amazing and so empowering. There was no fear and no more panic; just my husband and me birthing a baby together.

I can remember some kind of pep talk Scott started giving himself, but there really was hardly any time. "I can do this, I can do this," I heard him repeat. Well, I was already doing this and it was awesome! Our baby boy's head emerged with ease and with another push, he was in the hands of his adoring father. Things were so calm. Scott and our new baby boy just stared into each other's eyes. It's a moment Scott says he will cherish forever. It was an infinite bond; their sacred moment.

He quickly handed baby boy to me and I just held him close on my chest and cried. He was so beautiful, so perfect, and so alert. It was as if he was taking everything in and just looked around as if he were letting us know that we did well. I couldn't believe it. I had done it! I had the natural birth I had always dreamed of, though obviously different from how I had planned. Looking back, I realize those moments of sheer panic had been transition and a fear that the pain would get so much worse, but it never did.

Our living room suddenly started filling up with volunteer EMTs and police. We live in a small town and supposedly when they got this call, everyone wanted to respond. I guess it's not every day that a baby is born unplanned at home. Though our moment of bliss as we welcomed our baby boy was interrupted, no one can take away from those first treasured moments together. They announced the time of birth to be 4:01 a.m., just twenty minutes from the time I made the call to my midwife.

I always wonder if I suddenly felt such a wave of calm and reassurance during my birth because maybe my mom was looking out for me. It feels so nice to believe this; that she was there with me during this cherished time. Whatever it was, just validating this belief that my body knows exactly what it is meant to do is liberating. Although it was really far from the peaceful, water birth I had originally envisioned, I wouldn't change anything about it. We plan to have more children, and I no longer have any fear of childbirth. I know that next time around, if I am so lucky as to have a low risk pregnancy, I will be staying as far away from a hospital birth as possible. And Scott is already begging to deliver the next baby.

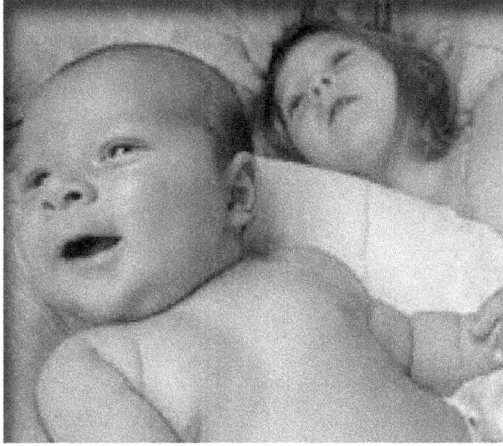

Micah and Ciela

With absolute love and joy, we welcomed:

Micah Travin Elliott

8 lbs 13 oz

21.5 inches

Born at home lovingly into the hands of his daddy.

Loved and cherished by all.

36

A Father's Take

By Scott Elliott

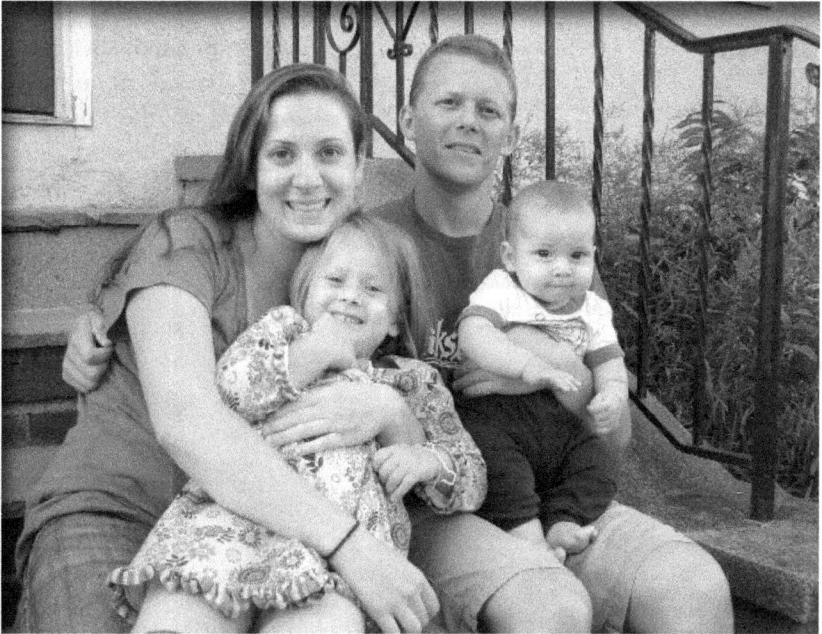

Elliott Family: Viviane, Scott, Ciela, and Micah

I was shot at, mortared, and on the receiving end of an IED during my time in Iraq. The initial moments of the unplanned home birth of my son were equally terrifying. Once I delivered him and determined that he was healthy, however, I came to love the intimacy of the home birth experience and vowed to deliver all of my future children in a similar, hospital-free manner.

It didn't sink in that I would have to deliver my son (I thought my wife was just being dramatic about her urgent need to give birth) until Viviane aimed her pelvis at my face and simply said, "Look." I was really glad this was my second child because if it were my first, I would not have understood what, exactly, I was looking at.

That's when I became truly afraid. Instincts took over and I simply coached Viviane through the pushing. On the edge of my consciousness, I imagined all of the things that could go wrong to prevent a successful birth. Deep down, beyond the chaos, I knew that everyone was going to be fine and that this was a great moment in our lives. It didn't take long before Viviane gave a final push and I caught Micah in my hands. The first thing he did was open his eyes, look deeply into mine, and take a breath. It was magical.

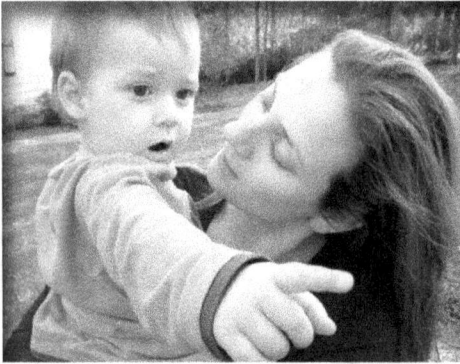

Viviane and Micah

I replay that moment a lot, and to this day, I still get goose bumps.

I was so proud of Viviane for being a good trooper and 'completing the mission,' regardless of the obstacles. I feel so thankful that Viviane and I shared this extremely bonding event; it was a moment of intimacy that few get to experience.

37

With My Own Two Hands

By Tiffany Burns

My journey to discovering the beauty and empowerment of natural childbirth began after the birth of my first child, Austin. My knowledge of childbirth, prior to his birth, came from the experiences of my close friends and family, which consisted only of obstetrician and hospital care. I followed the majority, which led to a "typical" hospital birth experience in our society today. Within five minutes of arriving at the hospital in labor with my first child, an electronic fetal monitor was strapped around my belly and an IV was in my arm administering fluids and penicillin (for Group B Strep). I was asked what my pain level was and if I would like an epidural. My intention was not to have an epidural, an intention that soon went south. I became nauseous within minutes of the penicillin being administered. I threw up more times than I can count. The nurse continually came in asking me if I was interested in the epidural. I finally took her up on the offer when she expressed concern with my son's heart beat dropping every time I vomited, and she thought the epidural would help. So there I was; IV in my arm, electronic fetal monitor around my belly, a barf bucket in my lap, and an epidural in my spine. Oh … and I almost forgot … a catheter. When it came time to push, I couldn't feel enough to even do so. I pushed for over an hour and a half when finally the obstetrician, who I had never met before, decided an episiotomy was necessary. I should state that I had never met any of the medical professionals involved in my care before that day (the nurse, nursing student, resident, or physician). My OB was part of a large group, so there was no guarantee he would deliver my son. In total, my labor was only a little over eight hours. I was absolutely in LOVE with my son at first sight, but the experience of labor was not pleasant and not something I wanted to repeat.

My realization that birth could be different was during an undergraduate ethics class. The class briefly went over some of the ethics regarding obstetrical care in our country and showed some clips from *The Business of Being Born*. Around this time my sister started to become interested in midwifery and we began bouncing ideas off of each other regarding birthing in this country.

Then during medical school, I took a medical humanities course called, "A Recent History of Childbirth." This was probably one of the best courses I took in my medical career. Along with a history of how modern obstetrics came to be, the class covered the current evidence-based medicine in childbirth. It was taught by a PhD who spent most of her career researching childbirth in our country compared to others. By the end of the class, I felt that if I wanted to have a natural, drug-free birth, my safest option would be to find a qualified midwife.

A few months after taking the class, my husband and I found out we were expecting again. We found a wonderful birth center not too far from our house that had two amazing, intelligent nurse midwives and one midwife in training. Since I knew pain meds were not going to be an option, I searched for birthing classes that could help keep me calm and get me through labor. I thankfully happened to stumble upon Hypnobabies. It is a childbirth program that completely re-defines the preconceived notions of childbirth that have been engrained into our subconscious since we were very young. It gives only positive affirmations surrounding childbirth. It suggests your birthing time will be easy, fast, and pain free. Yes, I said PAIN FREE. The mind is a powerful thing and pain is a matter of perception. Basically, the concept is a woman might experience pain because she is expecting childbirth to be painful and she is fearful of the pain. Anyway, once I stumbled upon Hypnobabies and I watched a few YouTube videos of Hypnobabies' births, I was sold!

On Saturday, January 29, 2011, I was studying all day for my renal domain exam. I was having some contractions, but I thought they were just toning contractions. They were nothing I couldn't study through. I felt great! My husband, Lucas, and our son, Austin, went to the local museum, and then went bowling. I stopped studying at 6:00 p.m. to clean the house because Lucas' brother and sister and their spouses were coming over to drop off some food for us. They came and we all had some good laughs. After they left, Lucas told me he was planning on taking Austin out to play with his cousin the next day. I wasn't happy about this because Lucas had been having a tendency to not answer his phone lately and my sister lives about 45 minutes away. I just felt like he needed to be close by. But he convinced me that he would keep his phone on him, and he told me, "You're going to be in labor at least two hours right. So that is plenty of time to get home to you if you need me." I agreed. We put Austin to bed and I called my sister Theresa to tell her that I had been having toning contractions all day. They weren't much, but I thought they might get stronger overnight. She said okay and that she would keep her phone by her. Lucas and I watched *Bones* and then I listened to my Hypnobabies "Visualize Your Birth" track on my iPod and fell asleep (I always fell asleep listening to my Hypnobabies tracks).

I slept great. I think listening to the Hypnobabies had something to do with it. I woke up at about **5:50 a.m.** to go to the bathroom. I had a contraction and noticed that I lost the rest of my mucus plug. I came back to bed and told Lucas I thought I was really in labor now. I had another contraction and used deep breathing to relax through it. I could feel it in my back, so I got on all fours to make myself more comfortable. Then I asked Lucas to heat up a rice sockie for me to put on my back. I also made him plug in my iPod to charge because I wanted to begin listening to my Hypnobabies "Birthing Day Affirmations," which would help me relax even more with each contraction. I told him, "Maybe I should call the Greenhouse Birth Center and just let them know I am in labor." He agreed. I called my little sister Theresa first; this was at **5:57 a.m.** I was planning on having her at the birth anyway, but she is also one of the post-partum doulas at the birth center. She asked if I wanted her to meet us at the birth center and I said I didn't know because I might just labor at home for a while until the contractions got stronger. Then I called the Greenhouse and left the message with the messaging center. A minute later (**6:05 a.m.**), Shelly, one of my midwives, who was already at the birth center because another mom was in labor there, called me back. Just as I answered the phone, I started to have another contraction. I told Shelly to wait one second. I got on my bed and breathed to relax and just allow the contraction to happen. After it was done I told Shelly what was going on. She thought I should come in and not wait too long. I told her I would take a shower and have Lucas get things together, and we would come in.

Lucas began to shave his face and gather the bags. I felt like I had to go pee again, so I sat on the toilet. Right then my water broke and I was having another contraction, but this time it was different. I felt some pressure. I reached down and I could feel my daughter's head. Lucas asked me if I wanted to just go right to the birth center. I said, **"No, she is coming now. Call Shelly back and bring me some towels."** He laid some towels down for me as he tried to call Shelly back. The line to the birth center was busy (Shelly said she was calling Clarice, the other midwife for back up since there was already one mom at the birth center). Lucas then called Theresa and told her to come to our house immediately or she was going to miss it.

She thought he was kidding (since he pranked her earlier in the week that I was in labor when I wasn't). Meanwhile, I could feel Lana's head moving down. I got down on my knees on the towels Lucas had just laid down for me. I didn't even have to push. My body was bearing down with the contraction. Lana slipped right out into *my own two hands*. I can't even begin to describe how amazing it was! She was perfect! Just prior to this (**6:10 a.m.**), Lucas had gone downstairs for something while on the phone, and finally got through to Shelly and told her we wouldn't be coming in. By the time he came back upstairs, he could hear Lana crying. He looked at me holding our little bundle and told Shelly, "Yup, she just had her." Shelly said when she heard her cry over the phone it was **6:12 a.m.** Lucas went and got baby blankets. Austin woke up and came into the bathroom. All smiles when he saw his baby sister. He said, **"MOM you squeezed your baby out!"** Then he came and sat by me. Lana started to nurse and we were as happy as could be. Theresa got there soon after and helped put some warm towels on me. Lucas made me breakfast … I was hungry! Shelly arrived and helped cut the cord and got me up and into bed. It was AMAZING! It was so calm and peaceful and everything I could have hoped for and more!

What a 180 from Austin's hospital birth! No drugs, no throwing up, no IV's or epidural. No heart rate monitors … no lying on my back in the worst position to push for over an hour and NO episiotomy! I couldn't have asked for more. I could move around (the greatness of not having local anesthetic)! And my bottom wasn't in pain from an episiotomy

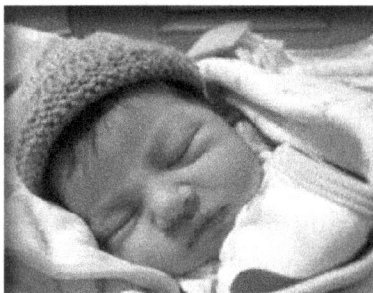

Lana

tear. What a difference not having those two interventions! I got to get right back into the comfort of my own bed with my baby. No having to pack up into a vehicle or move from place to place. Lana was measured and weighed right in bed with me. She was 7 lbs 8 oz and 20.5 inches long. The comfort of my own house was amazing. My wonderful sister helped me take an amazing herbal bath with Lana a few hours after she was born, and I was able to take a shower and get dressed.

And yes, I did have a PAIN FREE birth! It was not discomfort free, but I would not describe any part of it as painful. It was actually the best experience of my life. I was relaxed and calm, but my endorphins must have been in full swing. The feeling of delivering my daughter *with my own two hands* was the most empowering and indescribably wonderful experience of my life!

$$38$$

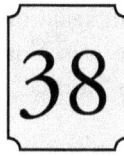

The Shocking Surprises of my Third Pregnancy

By Christina Mroz

The story of my third pregnancy is very unique. So, let me start at the beginning. Four months after my son, Kaleb, was born I started ovulating. Same thing happened after the birth of my daughter. My husband, Mike, and I decided to try natural family planning; although we were pretty sure we were done having children. One day, I realized that I was a couple of days late in menstruating. I mentioned this to Mike. That night he did not sleep well because he kept wondering if I might be pregnant. (It is very unusual for me to be late; my cycle tends to run like clockwork.) The very next day, he purchased a pregnancy test. Prior to taking it, I really didn't think I was pregnant. So next came the results ... yep, I was pregnant. Shock #1. It took me several days to let it all sink in. And it took me even longer to accept God's plan for my life. I remember calling my friend, Brooke, and just sobbing, and then I felt guilty for sobbing.

See, I'm a person who needs to have control. Both my daughter, Hannah, and my son, Kaleb, were planned down to the day, and it only took one try for us to conceive. I knew what worked best in my schedule and with my plans, but now God had totally messed with everything. After several months, I was finally able to accept the new responsibility that God had placed in my life.

I also struggled with the aspect of being pregnant again so soon. After four months, I finally felt like I was getting back to normal. I was back to my original weight. I was getting back into my yoga practice. I was looking forward to a little more freedom and a little more sleep. I was also not mentally prepared to be pregnant again or to give birth again—it was still all too fresh in my mind from my son. Not that my experience with my son was bad, but I just wanted to be "normal" for a little bit longer.

We did not tell our families for quite a while because we were adjusting to the idea of a third child ourselves. Our son would be only 14 months old when this baby arrived. We finally told our family through a picture. Hannah drew a picture of our family, and then she drew an extra person. I labeled them all, and then put ??? next to the fifth person. Our family was totally shocked. Shock #2. When we started telling people, they were shocked as well. Shock #3. I had several people say, "Aren't you still breastfeeding?" And I would answer, "Yes, but you can still get pregnant." I was amazed at how many people still think you can't get pregnant if you are nursing. I nursed my daughter until she was about 14 months old. However, with my son I barely made it to six months. Nursing and being pregnant was draining my entire body. I physically could no longer do it. Another thing out of my control—not my plan.

My first two labors were really fast. One was six hours and the second was five hours. I had both of these births at Morning Star Birth Center in Menomonie, WI. I loved the care there, I loved my birth experiences; however, I really wanted to try a home birth this time. Unfortunately, I lived outside Morning Star's radius for home births. So that led me to search for a new midwife that would do a home birth. This is when I came across Women Care from Winona, MN. Mike and I met with LeAnn and Brenda and decided this would be a perfect fit.

My entire pregnancy was very similar to my other ones. I didn't experience any morning sickness, I was gaining the same amount of weight, and I didn't have weird cravings. At my first prenatal, we noticed I was a little bit bigger than my projected number of weeks pregnant. However, I had only cycled twice prior to conceiving, so we weren't sure if I was on a 28, 29, 30, 31, or 32 day cycle. Therefore, my due date was always a little questionable. We finally settled on February 18th, 2011. LeAnn did discuss having an ultrasound done, so we could more accurately nail down my due date. However, we have never had an ultrasound done with our pregnancies and didn't feel the need to really nail down the due date. We felt that the baby would come when it would come. And, we felt that no matter what abnormality an ultrasound showed us that we would still love and care for this child in the same way, so why get one done. Now this is an area of control I didn't struggle with. I didn't need to know that everything was 100% okay, and I didn't need to know what the sex of the baby was either.

At about week 36, I mentioned that I felt a lot bigger. My maternity clothes were no longer fitting, so I was wearing Mike's shirts. My fundal height was only 1 to 2 cm different than with my other kids. However, my circumference was a lot different. At 37 weeks, I measured my waist at 42 inches. I was 39 inches with my other two kids the day I went into labor (and with both of them I went two days overdue). Everyone just kept telling me that a person is bigger with their third pregnancy.

On the mornings of February 1st and 2nd, I started to have some irregular contractions. I only had sporadic contractions for a couple of hours in the morning on these days, and then they would go away after lunch. I thought I was experiencing early labor, which I never experienced with my first two pregnancies. My girlfriend, Stephanie, had experienced early labor for weeks with her third child. I emailed her and told her what I was experiencing. She said she would start praying for me now because early labor was very frustrating and exhausting for her.

On the morning of February 3rd, I had to teach a Fit City class (an exercise class for people 55 and older), I just prayed that I didn't have contractions like the previous mornings. Interestingly enough, I did not. That evening, I had just gotten home from running some errands in town and was playing games with my daughter and husband when I had a couple of contractions— very similar to the ones I had the previous mornings. This was about 6:15 p.m. At 6:30 p.m., we were downstairs watching *Wheel of Fortune* and the contractions were coming on a regular basis, but they weren't very long. Mike asked if I was okay and I said yes. At 6:55 p.m., we decided to call LeAnn and let her know I was having contractions. We decided to start timing the contractions, and LeAnn said she would get back to us in a little while. The timing of the contractions was all over the board. Some contractions would only last 30 seconds, and then the next would be over a minute, and then they would be back down to 30 seconds. They were only a couple of minutes apart though.

Now, I need to set the stage for what was also happening during all of this. Both of our children were up, and Kaleb was getting a little testy because he was tired. Our pellet stove had just gone out and Mike needed to clean it before he could start it again. Now this might not seem like a big deal, but our bedroom is downstairs and often very cold. The pellet stove is essential to heating our room, and our bedroom is the room I planned to birth in. We also needed to start getting things ready for the home birth if I really was in labor, which meant changing sheets and getting out our supplies.

At about 7:15 p.m., Kaleb wanted me to cuddle him, but I didn't even want him around me. Mike decided to take him upstairs to bed. Normally, he goes to bed at 8 p.m. Hannah kept asking me if I was okay, and we just said "Momma might be having a baby tonight." A few minutes after this, Mike started stripping the bed and I walked into our bedroom to help. I had a few contractions while lying in bed; they seemed to be getting more intense, but not necessarily longer than before. At 7:25 p.m., I told Mike to call LeAnn because she needed to be here. Immediately after this, I was standing up near our bed and had a huge contraction. During this contraction, it almost felt like I needed to push (I think I did push a little) and my water broke. I was still wearing all my clothes and was afraid I was going to get the rug under our bed wet, so I started to move off the rug. I told Mike I had to go to the bathroom, which was just a couple feet away from our bed. (I didn't mention to him that I felt like I had to push—because that just seemed a little crazy.) I was just about to go to the restroom when I had another contraction. This time I stood up and said, "Mike, the baby is coming." I reached down and felt the head and gently glided the baby out. Mike immediately grabbed a towel and the baby started to cry. He also got some blankets wrapped around me as I sat on the toilet. Because of the coolness of the bathroom, he had to get our space heater, and he cranked it up. Shock #4—I just delivered my baby all by myself.

Mike immediately got on the phone with LeAnn to find out what we should do. Now, we did have a sheet titled "What if your midwives don't make it," but do you think either of us thought to look at the sheet—of course not. LeAnn said to keep the baby warm, skin-to-skin, and just wait until someone got there. However, the baby's umbilical cord was rather short and I couldn't bring it up to my torso, so just blankets had to do. After a couple of minutes I said to Mike, "I wonder what time the baby was born?" (Thanks to cell phone logs, we were able to go back through the phone calls exchanged and find out the time of the baby's birth—7:31 p.m.) I sat on the toilet for what seemed like forever. Mike called LeAnn again to ask about the placenta. He wanted to know what he was supposed to do if I delivered it. She told him to catch it. During this call, I started to have a contraction and I stood up so Mike could get the placenta. However, when Mike felt it something didn't seem right. And then came Shock #5— the biggest of them all. Mike was still on the phone (but by this time he had set it on the floor), "It is another baby." So Mike delivered baby number 2. I sat back down on the toilet holding not one, but now two babies who were wrapped in towels. Mike and I were just stunned. We had NO idea we were having twins. As I waited, I just had to call someone because NO one was going to believe this story. I called my mom. I basically said something like this, "Mom, I don't have a lot of time. I went into labor. Our midwives didn't make it, so I delivered the baby. And then Mike delivered the second baby. We had twins. (She started crying.) I am not joking. I'm totally serious. Please call Mikes' parents for us. We are all fine, we are just waiting for the midwives. We will call again soon." Shock #6!!! A couple minutes later, Mike started getting some texts from his dad.

Hannah was around during all of this. We can't remember exactly what she was doing, but she was around. We did ask her to get some towels for us, which she did. I also remember that when I was holding them she wanted to touch the babies, but was afraid. We just assured her that she could touch them, which she did. At this point, I wasn't even sure if they were boys or girls, but Mike said they were both girls. Thank goodness one of them was a girl because Hannah wanted a sister so bad!

For about 10 minutes, I just sat on the toilet with the babies. I couldn't move anywhere until the placenta was out. This is when someone came into our house. We figured it was LeAnn, but the strange thing was—the person was taking their "sweet" time. Mike finally went upstairs and noticed it was Erica, the birth assistant. Mike finally said, "She is on the toilet downstairs," as she handed him her coffee. As Erica came into my view, she stopped in her tracks. Shock # 7—she had no idea that I had delivered the baby myself, and she didn't know that I had delivered two babies. Our midwife had not been able to tell her prior to her arrival at our house. Erica came into the bathroom and chatted with us awhile and made sure we were all okay, which we were. At about 8:00 p.m., I birthed the placenta and Erica caught it in a bowl. That is when we moved to the bed. We made sure the girls didn't get mixed up, which was a concern of ours. Next, LeAnn showed up and was able to cut the umbilical cords. Upon cutting them, we discussed how we were going to tell them apart. Marker on the foot was discussed, but then Erica mentioned painting one of their toenails, which is what we did. The girl with the painted toe ended up being Elsa Lynn Mroz, born at 7:31 p.m. weighing 5 pounds, 10.5 ounces and was 18 ¾ inches long. The girl without the painted toe was … we weren't sure, we didn't

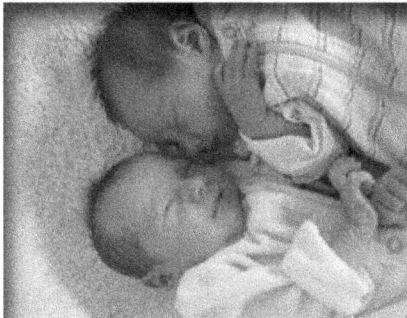

Elsa and Ellianna

have a second girl's name. The only other name I liked was Ellianna, so we decided to go with that. Then they asked how we would spell it, I got a piece of paper and wrote out four different spellings, and then Mike and I chose one. Next was the middle name, we had nothing. I told Mike it needed to be short and he said Ruth. Perfect, Ruth is my grandmother's first name. So the girl without her toe painted was Ellianna Ruth born at 7:41 p.m. weighing 5 pounds 13.5 ounces and was 19 inches long.

At one point during the exam of the babies, Hannah came downstairs with a grapefruit and said, "I brought a grapefruit for the babies to eat." It was so cute. She went to bed at about 9:15 p.m. because she was getting a little too crazy and was a bit overtired.

I can't remember when, but our second midwife showed up sometime. She came all the way from Iowa and was pulled over twice by cops on the way to my house. She got off both times—they actually believed her story.

Around 11 p.m., I had an herbal bath with both of the girls. My midwifery team commented that there was no clean up—which was very rare. But they did clean my bathroom and put a load of towels in the washer for us. At 11:45 p.m., our midwifery team all said good night and departed our house. Mike and I were now proud parents of not one, but two baby girls.

My friend, Megan, left me a voicemail that said, "I think Jesus is smiling a little bit." And she mentioned that it might have been a blessing that I didn't know I was having twins. She was right on both accounts. Yes, Jesus was smiling because he really is in control—not me. And yes, had I known I was having twins I probably would have thrown myself a huge pity party.

As I finish this really LONG story you probably have some questions.

How did we not know we were having twins? We never got an ultrasound to start. Second, we never noticed Ellianna. Elsa was the one the midwives always felt and the heartbeat we always heard. She was basically hiding Ellianna. Also, we discovered based on how they were born that both of the babies' hands and feet faced my spine. Now it made total sense why I never felt little feet or hands like I did with my first two pregnancies. The only thing that was unusual was my waist circumference. I also had this weird lump right under my ribcage that we could never quite figure out, but the midwives thought it was a knee. It was really the back of Ellianna's head. (Both of my midwives had never misdiagnosed twins before.) I do remember looking at Elsa when she was first born and thinking she was tiny—Mike even said the same thing. No wonder I didn't feel the "ring of fire," like I had with my other two births. Also, I remember glancing at my belly once and thinking ... boy it is still pretty rounded, I thought it would be more flat and squishy.

Were you scared? Not at all. I have never been afraid of birth. I've always known it is something I can do. The only time Mike and I were a little concerned was when Ellianna was first born, she didn't cry right away, but she did after about 30 seconds.

There really is not a way to end a story like this but to say … God is totally in control of my life—I totally got the message, God! And, this is one heck of a story!

Final Thoughts

Birthing takes courage of many kinds—courage to trust others, courage to make choices that might not always please our loved ones, courage to overcome our fears, courage to face the unknown, courage to say *no* when it is necessary. These stories and the additional planning information included in this book are meant to encourage and inspire women who desire to birth naturally, not as a means to pass judgment on those who do not. No matter what kind of birth a woman chooses, she will need courage and she can always use support.

It is my great hope that this book will inspire women to think about their birth choices, to heed their birthing instincts, and to commit themselves to the incredible physical and mental challenge that birth truly is.

Bibliography

American Association of Birth Centers. (2010). *What is a birth center? Membership Directory 2010.* Perkiomenville, PA: The American Association of Childbearing Centers.

Balaskas, J. (1992). *Active birth: the new approach to giving birth naturally.* Revised edition. Boston, MA: The Harvard Common Press.

Block, J. (2007). *Pushed: the painful truth about childbirth and modern maternity care.* Philadelphia, PA: DeCapo Press.

Centers for Disease Control and Prevention. (2010). *Births: Preliminary data for 2010: Maternal and infant health birth characteristics,* 5. Retrieved January 8, 2012, from http://www.cdc.gov/nchs/data/nvsr/nvsr60/nvsr60_02.pdf.

Connecticut Childbirth & Women's Center. (2006). *Who is a certified nurse-midwife?* Retrieved on January 5, 2012. http://www.ctbirthcenter.com/index.htm.

England, P. and Horowitz, R. (1998). *Birthing from within.* Albuquerque, NM: Partera Press.

Gaskin, I. M. (2011). *Birth matters: A midwife's manifesta.* New York: NY: Seven Stories Press.

Gaskin, I. M. (2003). *Ina May's guide to childbirth.* New York, NY: Bantam Books.

Gaskin, I.M. (1990). *Spiritual midwifery.* Summertown, TN: The Book Company.

Goer, H. (1995). *Obstetric myths versus research realties: A guide to the medical literature.* Westport, CT: Bergin & Garvey.

Goer, H. (1999). *The thinking woman's guide to a better birth.* New York, NY: A Perigee Book.

Greene, M. F. (2004). Vaginal birth after cesarean revisited. *New England Journal of Medicine 351* (25), 2647-2649.

Katz-Rothman, B. (2011). Barbara Katz Rothman. Retrieved on 8/14/11 from www.barbarakatzrothman.com.

Landon, M. (2004). Maternal and perinatal outcomes associated with a trial of labor with previous cesarean section. *New England Journal of Medicine, 351*(25), 2655-2659.

Mallak, J., & Bailey, T. (2010). *The doulas' guide to birthing your way*. Amarillo, TX: Hale Publishing.

MacDorman, M.F., Declercq, E., & Mathews, T.J. (2011). United States home births increase 2 percent from 2004 to 2004. *Birth, 38* (3), 185–190. Retrieved January 8, 2012 from http://onlinelibrary.wiley.com/doi/10.1111/j.1523-536X.2011.00481.x/abstract.

Midwives Alliance of North America. (2011). *Direct-entry midwife (DEM)*. Retrieved January 5, 2012, from http://mana.org/definitions.html.

Mongan, M. F. (2005). *Hypnobirthing: the Mongan method*. Third edition. Deerfield Beach, FL: Health Communications, Inc.

Sears, W., & Sears, M. (1994). *The birth book: everything you need to know to have a safe and satisfying birth*. New York, NY: Little, Brown and Company.

Simkin, P. (2008). *The birth partner: A complete guide to childbirth for dads, doulas, and all other labor companions*. Third edition. Boston, MA: The Harvard Common Press.

Simkin, P., & Ancheta, R. (2011). *The labor progress handbook: Early interventions to prevent and treat dystocia* (3rd ed.). Oxford, UK: Wiley-Blackwell.

Wagner, M. (2006). *Born in the USA: How a broken maternity system must be fixed to put mothers and infants first*. Berkeley, CA: University of California Press.

Recommended Reading

Arms, S.(1996). *Immaculate deception II: Myth, magic & birth.* Berkeley, CA: Celestial Arts.

Balaskas, J. (1992). *Active birth. The new approach to giving birth naturally* (Rev. ed.). Boston, MA: Harvard Common Press.

Block, J. (2008). *Pushed: The painful truth about childbirth and modern maternity care.* Cambridge, MA: Da Capo Press.

Buckley, S. J. (2008). *Gentle birth, gentle mothering.* Berkeley, CA: Celestial Arts.

Davis-Floyd, R. (2004). *Birth as an American rite of passage: Second edition.* Los Angeles, CA: University of California Press.

Dick-Read, G., & Odent, M. (2005). *Childbirth without fear: The principles and practice of natural childbirth.* London: Pinter & Martin Ltd.

England, P., & Horowitz, R. (1998). *Birthing from within: An extra-ordinary guide to childbirth preparation.* Albuquerque, NM: Partera Press.

Gaskin, I.M. (2011). *Birth matters: A midwife's manifesta.* New York, NY: Seven Stories Press.

Gaskin, I.M. (2003). *Ina May's guide to childbirth.* New York, NY: Bantam.

Gaskin, I.M. (2002). *Spiritual midwifery.* Summertown, TN: Book Publishing Co.

Goer, H. (1995). *Obstetric myths versus research realities: A guide to the medical literature.* Westport, CT: Bergin & Garvey.

Goer, H. (1999). *The thinking woman's guide to a better birth.* New York, NY: Perigee Trade.

Harper, B., & Arms, S. (2005). *Gentle birth choices.* Rochester, VT: Healing Arts Press.

Kitzinger, S. (2003). *The complete book of pregnancy and childbirth.* New York: Alfred A. Knopf.

Korte, D. (1997). *The VBAC companion.* Boston, MA: Harvard Common Press.

Lothian, J., & De Vries, C. (2010). *The official Lamaze guide: Giving birth with confidence (2nd ed.).* Minnetonka, MN: Meadowbrook Press.

Mallak, J.S., & Bailey, T.F. (2010). *The doulas' guide to birthing your way.* Amarillo, TX: Hale Publishing.

Mongan, M.F. (2005). *Hypnobirthing: The Mongan method: A natural approach to a safe, easier, more comfortable birthing.* 3rd ed. Deerfield Beach, FL: Health Communications.

Odent, M. (1994). *Birth reborn.* Medford, NJ: Birth Works.

Odent, M. (2004). *The Cesarean.* London: Free Association Books.

Panuthos, C. (1984). *Transformation through birth.* Bergin & Garvey.

Rothman, B.K. (1991). *In labor: Women and power in the birthplace.* New York, NY: W.W. Norton & Co. Inc.

Sears, W., & Sears, M. (1994). *The birth book: Everything you need to know to have a safe and satisfying birth.* New York: Little, Brown and Company.

Simkin, P. (2008). *The birth partner: A complete guide to childbirth for dads, doulas, and all other labor companions* (Rev. 3rd ed.). Boston, MA: Harvard Common Press.

Simkin, P., & Ancheta, R. (2011). *The labor progress handbook: Early interventions to prevent and treat dystocia* (3rd ed.). West Sussex, UK: Wiley-Blackwell.

Tupler, J., & Thompson, A. (1996). *Maternal fitness: Preparing for a healthy pregnancy, an easier labor, and a quick recovery.* New York, NY: Touchstone.

Wagner, M. (2008). *Born in the USA: How a broken maternity system must be fixed to put women and children first.* Los Angeles, CA: University of California Press.

Essential Planning Directory

If you are planning to birth naturally, you will find the following resources helpful in finding the right care provider, support, and information to get you ready.

American Association of Birth Centers (AABC)

(866) 54BIRTH

www.birthcenters.org

American College of Nurse-Midwives (ACNM)

(888) MIDWIFE

www.midwife.org

Birthing from Within

(805) 964-6611

www.birthingfromwithin.com

Birthing the Future

(970) 884-4005

www.birthingthefuture.org

Birthworks

(888) 862-4784

www.birthworks.org

Bradley Method of Natural Childbirth

(800) 4-A-BIRTH

www.bradleybirth.com

Childbirth and Postpartum Professionals Association (CAPPA)

(888) MY-CAPPA

www.cappa.net

DONA International

(888) 788-DONA (3662)

www.dona.org

HypnoBabies

(714) 952-BABY

www.hypnobabies.com

HypnoBirthing

(603) 798-4781

www.hypnobirthing.com

International Birth and Wellness Project (ALACE)

(877) 334-4297

www.alace.org

International Cesarean Awareness Network (ICAN)

(800) 686-ICAN

www.ICAN-Online.org

International Childbirth Education Association, Inc. (ICEA)

(800) 624-4934
www.ICEA.org

La Leche League

(800) LALECHE
www.lalecheleague.org

Lamaze International

(800) 368-4404
www.lamaze.org

Midwifery Today

www.midwiferytoday.com

Midwives Alliance of North America (MANA)

(888) 923-MANA
www.mana.org

Postpartum Support International

(800) 944-4PPD
www.postpartum.net

Glossary

Active phase of labor: This phase begins around 3–5 centimeters dilation. At this point labor begins to become more intense.

Acupressure: Also known as shiatsu, a means to relieve pain during labor in which fingers apply pressure to various pain-controlling points on the body.

Amniotic fluid: Fluid that is produced by the water bag during pregnancy.

Amniotomy: Also known as rupturing the membranes. During this procedure your midwife or doctor will insert an amniohook into the vagina and gently snag the membranes, breaking the bag of waters.

Antepartum: Before labor

Apgar Score: A means of assessing the well being of a new born by scoring the heart rate, color, muscle tone, respiration ability and reactivity. Scores range from 0—10. A score of 7 or lower at five minutes after birth indicates a need for medical attention.

Bradley method: Husband coached natural childbirth preparatory course

Braxton-Hicks Contractions: Non-labor, painless contractions

Certified nurse-midwife: An educated and licensed practitioner in the two disciplines of nursing and midwifery. She must pass a national certification examination given by the American College of Nurse-Midwives and must meet strict requirements set forth by (her state's) Department of Public Health.

Cervidil (dinoprostone): A prostaglandin suppository used to artificially stimulate cervix ripening

Cervix: The narrow passage forming the lower end of the uterus.

Cytotec: A drug often used as a "cervical ripener" or to induce labor. It has been known to cause uterine rupture, injury, or death to mother or baby. The generic name for Cytotec is Misoprostrol.

Dilation: Opening of the cervix

Direct-entry midwife: An independent practitioner educated in the discipline of midwifery through self-study, apprenticeship, a midwifery school, or a college—or university—based program distinct from the discipline of nursing. A direct-entry midwife is trained to provide the Midwives Model of Care to healthy women and newborns throughout the childbearing cycle, primarily in out-of-hospital settings.

Doula: A labor companion. May be trained or not trained.

Dystocia: A birth that is difficult and slow to progress.

Effacement: Thinning of the cervix.

Endorphins: Chemicals produced in the pituitary gland and the hypothalamus and released during labor, which help woman cope with the intensity of the contractions and feel good.

Epidural: Anesthesia placed in the space near the spine through a catheter.

Episiotomy: An incision on the perineum to enlarge the opening of the vagina during childbirth.

Group B Strep or Group Beta Strep: A bacterium that can colonize in the female reproductive tract and can possibly cause pneumonia or meningitis in newborns.

Hydrotherapy: Use of water during labor to ease intensity.

Hypnobabies: A program of hypnosis for childbirth developed by Kerry Tuschhoff.

HypnoBirthing: A course in hypnosis for childbirth developed by Marie Mongan.

ICAN (International Cesarean Awareness Network): A national organization offering support groups, information, and healing for women planning VBAC.

Induction: Forcing labor to begin before it begins spontaneously.

Kegel exercise: Pelvic-floor strengthening exercise - controlled tightening of the muscles in the vagina and rectum. This exercise helps women prepare for birth and regain muscle function after birth.

Latent phase of labor: Early labor. Usually not very intense.

Lightening: When the baby drops lower in preparation for birth.

Mantra: A word or short phrase that you can repeat to help keep yourself concentrating on your goal.

Meconium: The first poop of a newborn. Meconium is very dark—almost black—sticky, and odorless.

Mucus plug: An accumulation of mucus in the cervix which helps protect the baby from infection. The mucus plug sometimes comes out right before labor begins.

Nipple stimulation: Causes the release of oxytocin, which sometimes initiates or strengthens labor rushes, can be accomplished manually or by using a breast pump.

Oxytocin: A hormone naturally released during labor, which causes contractions and initiates milk production after birth.

Perineum: The skin and muscle that is between the bottom of the vagina and the rectum.

Pitocin: Synthetic oxytocin used to induce or enhance labor, also used to stop bleeding after birth.

Placenta: Also known as the afterbirth, this is an organ that transfers nutrients, oxygen, hormones, and waste between mother and baby.

Postpartum doula: A trained individual who assists the new mother after the birth of the baby.

Pre-eclampsia: A disease that sometimes occurs during pregnancy. Symptoms include high blood pressure, protein in the urine, and swelling.

Prostaglandins: Naturally or artificially occurring substances that help the cervix ripen. Semen is a natural prostaglandin.

Rebozo: A shawl used by midwives to help position the baby during labor.

Rushes: A gentler term for contractions.

Sterile water injection: Injection of sterile water into the dimples on the small of your back. The water creates a stinging sensation, which activates the release of endorphins, easing the pain in that area.

Stripping or sweeping the membranes: A finger inserted inside the vagina during a pelvic exam by the doctor or midwife to separate the amniotic sac from the uterus. This process often triggers labor.

Transition: The period the cervix completes dilation from 8 - 10 centimeters. This is the last and most intense part of active labor. Transition can last from a few minutes to around an hour.

Uterine rupture: The opening of a uterine scar that poses a serious health risk to mother and baby.

VBAC: Vaginal birth after Cesarean.

Index

About the Author

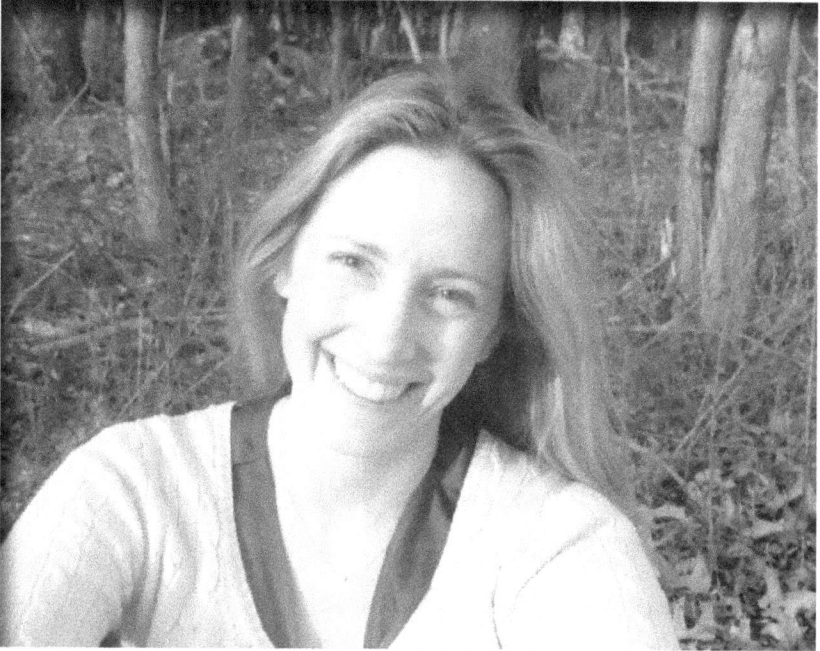

Natasha Panzer is a mother, wife, writer, teacher, and natural birth advocate. She was inspired to create this book after the incredible natural water birth of her second child.

Natasha earned her bachelor's degree for Dramatic Writing from the Tisch School of the Arts at New York University. She earned her master's degree for Teaching English as a Second Language from Western Connecticut State University. She lives in Dutchess County, New York, with her husband and two children. This is her first book.